YOGA
for you

Other titles in this series:

MOTORBIKE mechanics
YOUR CAR fault finder
What to FREEZE and how
How to play TENNIS
PHOTOGRAPHY made easy

YOGA
for you

Text by John Davis
Illustrations by Max Lenvers
with Brian Netscher

Series Editor P. Cassidy

Mirror Books

Published by Mirror Books Ltd.,
Athene House, 66/73 Shoe Lane,
London EC4P 4AB
for Mirror Group Newspapers Ltd.

© Chancerel Publishers Ltd., 1980
Paperback edition June 1980

Produced for Mirror Books Ltd by
Chancerel Publishers Ltd.,
40 Tavistock Street,
London WC2E 7PB.

ISBN 0 85939 213 9

Origination by ReproSharp, London EC1.

Printed in Great Britain by
Richard Clay (The Chaucer Press) Ltd.,
Bungay, Suffolk, England.

CONTENTS

Chapter 1

WHAT IS YOGA?

Over the past hundred years, people in the West have looked to the East to see if something can be learned from the ancient Eastern philosophies. Today even more, people look to the Eastern philosophies as a way of obtaining peace of mind and calm in a high-speed world, full of stresses and strains. Yoga is one of these philosophies, which has attracted great interest everywhere.

Yoga is not a religion, but a discipline which helps man to become whole, at peace with himself, rather than a confusion of different parts — mind, body, emotions and spirit — all pulling in different directions. The word yoga comes from Sanskrit, an ancient and sacred language of India. It means to harness together. It contains the idea of union and mastery. Our English words 'join' and 'yoke' come from the same origin.

The best way to discover yoga is to try it yourself. People of all ages and walks of life can practise yoga and you don't need a lot of expensive equipment. Yoga is a kind of self-improvement course, affecting your physical and mental health. It increases your level of awareness and heightens your perceptions. A feeling of serenity develops, as the tensions of modern living are left behind.

Hatha Yoga

Hatha (physical) yoga is the yoga usually practised in the West and the one most people mean when they talk about yoga. Physical postures (asanas), relaxation, breathing and cleansing techniques are used to reach a state of physical and mental well-being. There are also techniques for improving concentration.

There are other kinds of yoga, of which the four main kinds are:

Raja Yoga teaches control of the mind and will. It has eight limbs or stages, of which Hatha Yoga is a part. The later stages lead further to deeper concentration, meditation and Samadhi, a state of union with the self, something like the Buddhist idea of Nirvana, a state of bliss in which the mind and body are one with the universe.

Karma Yoga teaches how to perform and enjoy the ordinary actions of life by serving others, without seeking reward or praise. It is the yoga of selfless actions in the world. Originally it meant sacrifice to the gods.

Jnana Yoga is for intellectuals, being the yoga of wisdom and knowledge. Jnana seeks the revelation of the Truth through deep understanding.

Bhakti Yoga is the yoga of devotion, involving faith and worship, concentration and meditation on the Absolute. It is known as the love of God.

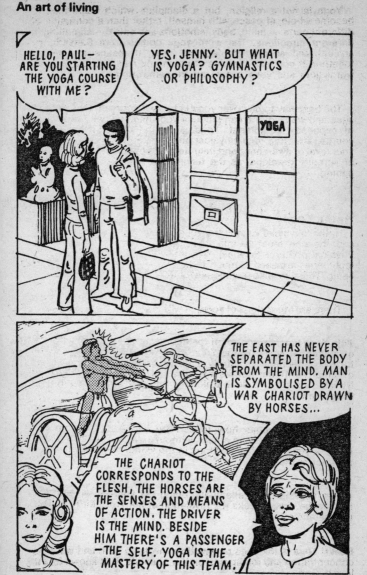

HELLO, PAUL— ARE YOU STARTING THE YOGA COURSE WITH ME?

YES, JENNY. BUT WHAT IS YOGA? GYMNASTICS OR PHILOSOPHY?

YOGA

THE EAST HAS NEVER SEPARATED THE BODY FROM THE MIND. MAN IS SYMBOLISED BY A WAR CHARIOT DRAWN BY HORSES...

THE CHARIOT CORRESPONDS TO THE FLESH, THE HORSES ARE THE SENSES AND MEANS OF ACTION. THE DRIVER IS THE MIND. BESIDE HIM THERE'S A PASSENGER —THE SELF. YOGA IS THE MASTERY OF THIS TEAM.

9

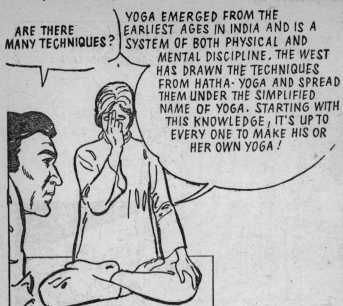

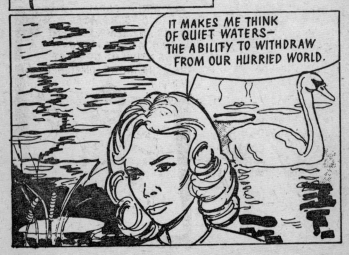

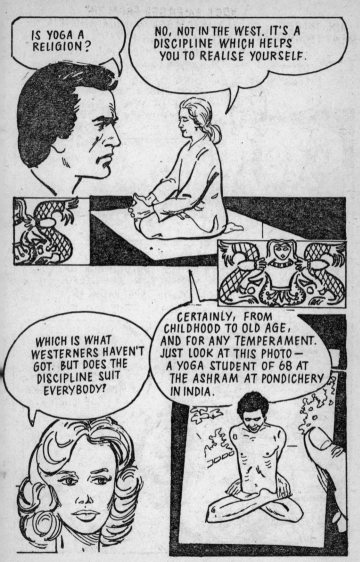

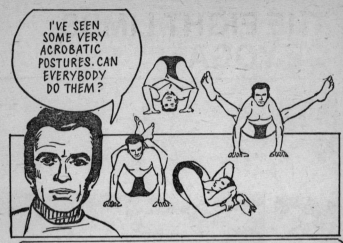

I'VE SEEN SOME VERY ACROBATIC POSTURES. CAN EVERYBODY DO THEM?

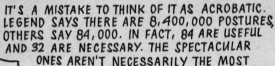

IT'S A MISTAKE TO THINK OF IT AS ACROBATIC. LEGEND SAYS THERE ARE 8,400,000 POSTURES, OTHERS SAY 84,000. IN FACT, 84 ARE USEFUL AND 32 ARE NECESSARY. THE SPECTACULAR ONES AREN'T NECESSARILY THE MOST EFFECTIVE.

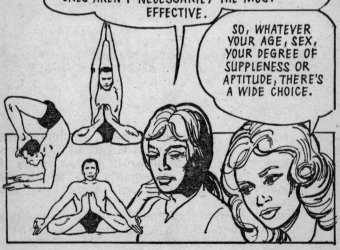

SO, WHATEVER YOUR AGE, SEX, YOUR DEGREE OF SUPPLENESS OR APTITUDE, THERE'S A WIDE CHOICE.

Chapter 2

THE EIGHT LIMBS OF YOGA

For countless generations yoga teaching was passed on by word of mouth. Then about 2000 years ago, a sage called Patanjali wrote down a series of aphorisms, or short statements, in which he explained the structure of yoga to his contemporaries.

Patanjali divided progress in yoga into eight stages, like the rungs of a ladder, and he called them the "Eight Limbs of Yoga".

First limb — Yama

Yama are restraints on behaviour, so that a person should not harm his fellow man. There are five: Ahimsa, non-violence; Satya, not lying; Asteya, not stealing; Brahmacharya, non-sensuality, temperance; and Aparigraha, not being mean.

Second limb — Niyama

Niyama is a positive concept. A person should observe certain ideas of discipline and adopt a joyful attitude to life. The five Niyama are: Shaucha, cleanliness, purity; Santosha, serenity, contentment; Tapas, austerity, discipline; Swadhyaya, general study and self examination; and Ishwara Pranidhana, devotion to an ideal.

In some ways the Yama and Niyama correspond to the Christian idea of the Ten Commandments, as rules of personal conduct.

Third limb — Asanas (postures)

Asanas are the physical movements or postures, which together with the fourth and fifth limbs, help the mind to withdraw from its constant preoccupation with the senses.

Fourth limb — Pranayama

Pranayama is breath control and exercises which are important in order to control and utilise the Prana (universal energy) with which every person is born.

Fifth limb — Pratyahara

Through concentrating the mind, the senses lose their importance and ability to influence a person's actions.

Sixth limb — Dharana

Fixing the attention on a single object helps to withdraw from the senses. Dharana means concentration.

Seventh limb — Dhyana

Meditation upon an object or idea.

Eighth limb — Samadhi

A state of union with the spiritual Self, like the Buddhist ideal of Nirvana. This is the ultimate goal of yoga.

The first five limbs of yoga are the external aspects of yoga, while the last three form the Samyama (holding together), which are the internal aspects of yoga, leading finally to absorption into the Absolute.

HATHA-YOGA PREPARES THE WAY TO RAJA-YOGA, OR ROYAL YOGA. BUT WESTERNERS DON'T ALL WANT TO SUBMIT THEMSELVES TO ITS INDISPENSABLE DISCIPLINE OF RESTRAINTS AND OBSERVANCES.

THESE ARE THE **YAMA** OR RESTRAINTS IN THOUGHT, WORD AND DEED: ONE SHOULD NOT WISH TO KILL OR STEAL, OR BE LUSTFUL, OR BE MISERLY. AVOID LYING.

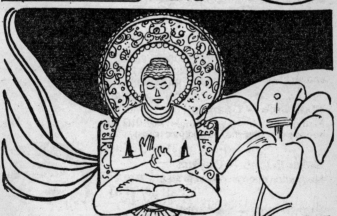

THESE ARE THE **NIYAMA** OR OBSERVANCES; TO PRACTISE PURIFICATION. TO BE JOYFUL. TO BE DISCIPLINED. TO STUDY THE GREAT SCRIPTURES. TO SEEK THE ABSOLUTE.

15

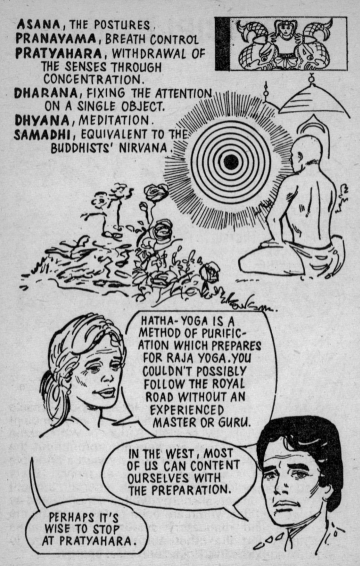

ASANA, THE POSTURES.
PRANAYAMA, BREATH CONTROL.
PRATYAHARA, WITHDRAWAL OF THE SENSES THROUGH CONCENTRATION.
DHARANA, FIXING THE ATTENTION ON A SINGLE OBJECT.
DHYANA, MEDITATION.
SAMADHI, EQUIVALENT TO THE BUDDHISTS' NIRVANA.

HATHA-YOGA IS A METHOD OF PURIFICATION WHICH PREPARES FOR RAJA YOGA. YOU COULDN'T POSSIBLY FOLLOW THE ROYAL ROAD WITHOUT AN EXPERIENCED MASTER OR GURU.

IN THE WEST, MOST OF US CAN CONTENT OURSELVES WITH THE PREPARATION.

PERHAPS IT'S WISE TO STOP AT PRATYAHARA.

Chapter 3

A PRINCIPLE OF LIFE

The roots of yoga lie in ideas about man's constitution which are found in a very ancient Eastern philosophy, called Samkya. With some variations these ideas are common throughout the East. It is a philosophy that puts forward a principle of life which is as much physical as mental. Every person comes into the world with a certain amount of Prana, or universal energy, which is maintained by the two systems which are open to the cosmos, the digestive and respiratory systems. One ensures breathing and the other nutrition. Yoga helps to control and preserve Prana, universal energy.

Breathing

Yoga regards breathing as more important than nutrition; as the primary source of Prana. Two of the main channels for Prana start at the nostrils, the Ida at the left nostril and the Pingala at the right.

When you breathe it is usually a completely automatic action, except when running a race or exerting yourself physically. By trying yoga breathing exercises you will notice how breathing operates on a conscious level. Normal breathing is shallow, only using the upper parts of the lungs. With breathing exercises you begin to breathe more deeply and learn how to control the way you breathe. Slow, rhythmic breathing makes you feel relaxed and helps avoid a build-up of tension.

Nutrition

Prana is also drawn from food. Some foods give energy and give a feeling of well-being and lightness, revitalising the system, while others leave a dull, heavy feeling, using more energy for digestion than is actually gained by eating them.

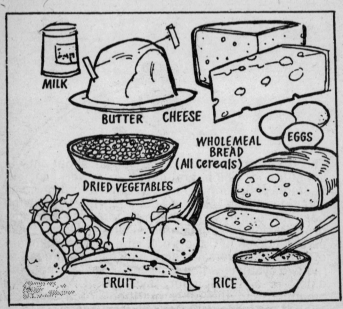

Some foods which give Prana

Fresh and lightly-cooked vegetables are good for you, also certain dried vegetables, which can be found in health food shops. Fruit, cheese, butter or margarine, wholemeal bread and all cereals, whole rice and milk are all excellent.

Refined sugar and flour products, high protein dishes, coffee, tea and alcohol may tend to deplete Prana. Meat, poultry and fish should be taken in moderate quantities. Foods which are tinned, preserved or processed should be avoided, also those with stimulants.

For most people these ideas should be taken as a guiding principle rather than a strict diet, as a sudden change to different eating habits or vegetarianism may be too radical after a lifetime of eating in one way. A gradual change to a lighter, healthier diet may be the best way. You will also find that regular work on postures and breathing exercises will reduce the amount of food you need to eat.

However much food you do eat, it is important to eat it properly. Eat slowly and chew food well before swallowing. Relax before you eat, so you can enjoy and appreciate the flavour of what you are eating.

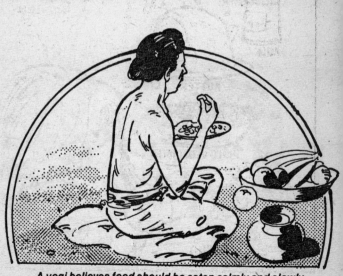

A yogi believes food should be eaten calmly and slowly.

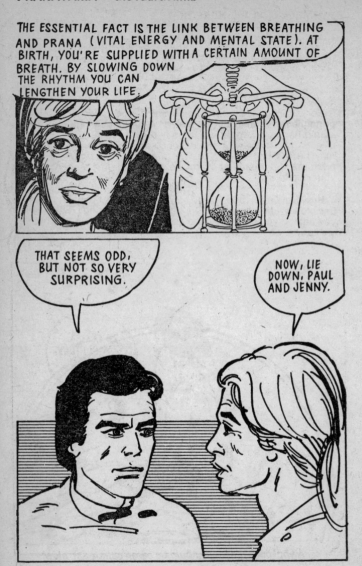

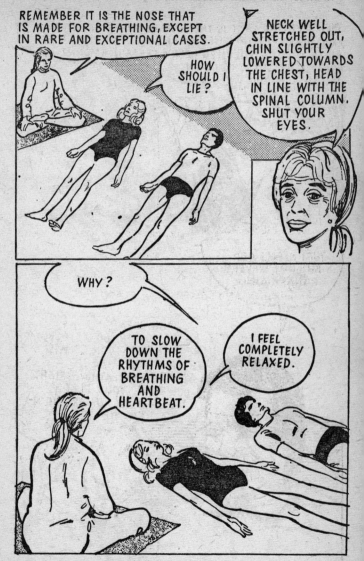

The three ways of breathing

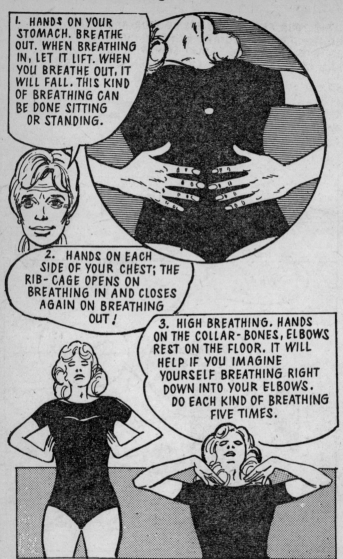

1. HANDS ON YOUR STOMACH. BREATHE OUT. WHEN BREATHING IN, LET IT LIFT. WHEN YOU BREATHE OUT, IT WILL FALL. THIS KIND OF BREATHING CAN BE DONE SITTING OR STANDING.

2. HANDS ON EACH SIDE OF YOUR CHEST; THE RIB-CAGE OPENS ON BREATHING IN AND CLOSES AGAIN ON BREATHING OUT!

3. HIGH BREATHING. HANDS ON THE COLLAR-BONES, ELBOWS REST ON THE FLOOR. IT WILL HELP IF YOU IMAGINE YOURSELF BREATHING RIGHT DOWN INTO YOUR ELBOWS. DO EACH KIND OF BREATHING FIVE TIMES.

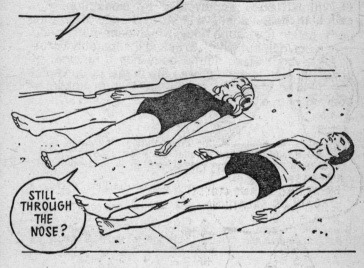

BRING YOUR ARMS DOWN BESIDE YOUR BODY, HANDS TURNED UPWARD. YOU ARE GOING TO COMBINE THE THREE KINDS OF BREATHING. START LOW WITH THE ABDOMEN, THEN THE MIDDLE OF THE CHEST, THEN THE TOP. SMOOTH AND SLOW. THAT'S RIGHT.

STILL THROUGH THE NOSE?

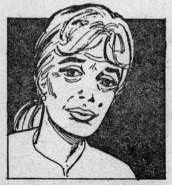

YES. OPEN THE NOSTRILS, BUT CONTRACT THE PHARYNX SLIGHTLY AND LET YOUR TONGUE LIE LIMP, OR COME UP A BIT OVER THE UPPER TEETH.

23

Chapter 4

THE TWO BODIES

In the West we tend only to believe in the things we can see. The anatomy we study in textbooks shows the human body as revealed by dissection. But people in the East believe in the existence of another body, called the subtle body, which cannot be found with a scalpel, but which is linked inseparably to the physical body. This subtle body has a network of channels along which moves the Prana, or universal energy. The channels, Nadis, are in turn linked to energy centres or Chakras.

Nadis

These are channels carrying Prana through the subtle body. They are comparable to the meridian lines used in Chinese acupuncture. There are thousands of Nadis in the subtle body, but the three main ones are:

Ida which starts at the left nostril and carries lunar energy, a negative current.

Pingala which starts at the right nostril and carries solar energy, a positive current.

Sushumna the central nadi, or nadi of fire, which corresponds to the spinal column and is the main channel for the flow of nervous energy.

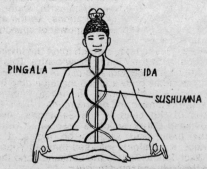

The main nadis — Ida, Pingala and Sushumna

Chakras

Chakras are part of the energy chain. Chakra means wheel in Sanskrit. The six main chakras act as centres of vital energy. Yogis, the devotees of yoga, see the chakras as being linked to a fine canal inside the spinal cord, and driven like imaginary turbine wheels by Ida and Pingala (negative and positive) currents to generate the physical and psychic energy necessary for life.

The five lower Chakras are said to influence the parts of the body in which they are situated, especially when energy is concentrated in that particular area through breath control or postures.

Starting at the base of the spine the first chakra is the Muladhara, which is linked to the element, earth, which gives earth qualities of weight and solidity. These in turn give rise to a feeling of security. The sense of smell is derived from the earth element. This chakra also controls the process of eliminating waste from the body.

The Muladhara contains a dormant power called Kundalini, or the Serpent power, which carries with it knowledge of good and evil when it is released. This energy should be used and controlled under the guidance of a teacher, as it controls the deepest aspects of the personality, the subconscious.

The second chakra, Svadhisthana, is associated with the element of water. One of the functions of fluid in the body is to produce saliva, so this chakra is connected with the sense of taste. It is also said to control sexual desire.

The third chakra, Manipura, situated on the level of the solar plexus on the spine, is associated with the element of fire. Fire gives heat and light, so this area is linked to the digestive processes (burning up food) and the sense of sight.

Anahata, the fourth chakra, is at the level of the heart. Its element is air which is connected to the sense of touch and the idea of human contact. This corresponds with our idea of the heart being involved in human relationships. This chakra controls breathing.

On a level with the throat and thyroid gland is the fifth chakra, Vishuddha, for which the element is space, called ether. Space contains the other four elements of earth, water, fire and air, which are all considered to be vibrations. As the ether contains them all, it is connected with sound (power of speech) which is the most powerful vibration.

The Vishuddha is the bridge which joins the lower elements to the idea of thought at the Ajna or brow centre. This is situated at the level of the pituitary gland. It is part of the endocrine system, which regulates all the body's functions, including the autonomic nervous system, which controls the involuntary action of the heart, lungs, liver, kidneys and other organs.

At the top of the head is the Sahasrara, also called the Thousand-petalled Lotus, which is associated with the cortical layer of the brain, and said to be the seat of Absolute Consciousness. Kundalini is released through Yoga and rises up the central Nadi, Sushumna, to the Sahasrara and the Yogi enters Samadhi as the body and mind merge.

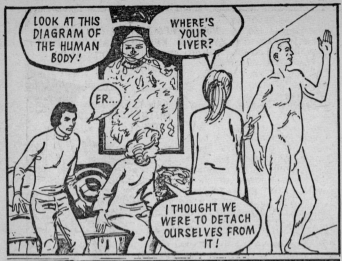

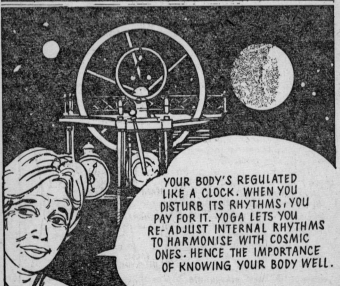

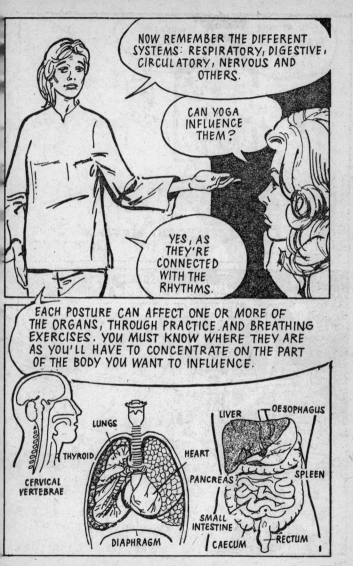

NOW REMEMBER THE DIFFERENT SYSTEMS: RESPIRATORY, DIGESTIVE, CIRCULATORY, NERVOUS AND OTHERS.

CAN YOGA INFLUENCE THEM?

YES, AS THEY'RE CONNECTED WITH THE RHYTHMS.

EACH POSTURE CAN AFFECT ONE OR MORE OF THE ORGANS, THROUGH PRACTICE AND BREATHING EXERCISES. YOU MUST KNOW WHERE THEY ARE AS YOU'LL HAVE TO CONCENTRATE ON THE PART OF THE BODY YOU WANT TO INFLUENCE.

CERVICAL VERTEBRAE

THYROID

LUNGS

HEART

DIAPHRAGM

LIVER

OESOPHAGUS

PANCREAS

SPLEEN

SMALL INTESTINE

CAECUM

RECTUM

27

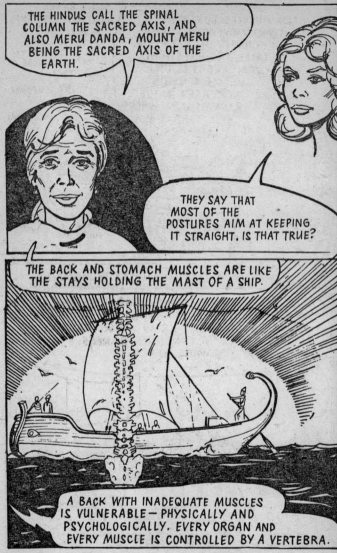

THE HINDUS CALL THE SPINAL COLUMN THE SACRED AXIS, AND ALSO MERU DANDA, MOUNT MERU BEING THE SACRED AXIS OF THE EARTH.

THEY SAY THAT MOST OF THE POSTURES AIM AT KEEPING IT STRAIGHT. IS THAT TRUE?

THE BACK AND STOMACH MUSCLES ARE LIKE THE STAYS HOLDING THE MAST OF A SHIP.

A BACK WITH INADEQUATE MUSCLES IS VULNERABLE — PHYSICALLY AND PSYCHOLOGICALLY. EVERY ORGAN AND EVERY MUSCLE IS CONTROLLED BY A VERTEBRA.

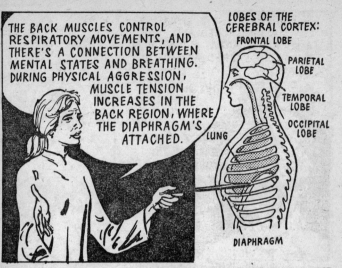

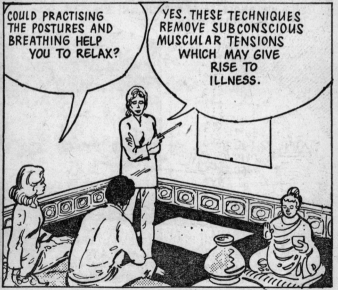

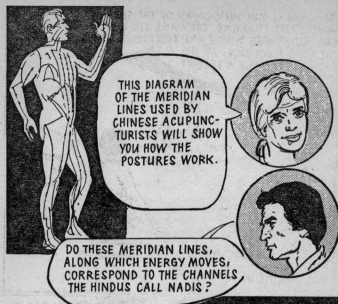

THIS DIAGRAM OF THE MERIDIAN LINES USED BY CHINESE ACUPUNCTURISTS WILL SHOW YOU HOW THE POSTURES WORK.

DO THESE MERIDIAN LINES, ALONG WHICH ENERGY MOVES, CORRESPOND TO THE CHANNELS THE HINDUS CALL NADIS?

ACCORDING TO SOME PEOPLE THERE ARE 72,000 NADIS, OTHERS SAY 360,000. IN ANY CASE THE DISTRIBUTION OF ENERGY (PRANA) WORKS ON THE SAME PRINCIPLE.

The Chakras

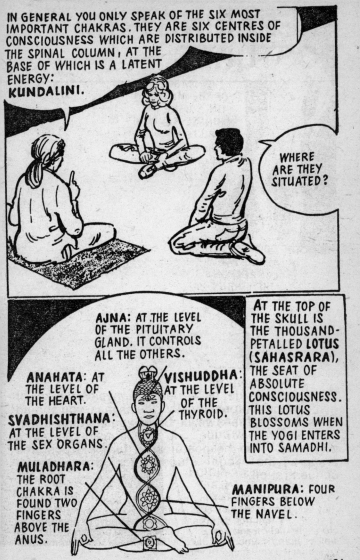

IN GENERAL YOU ONLY SPEAK OF THE SIX MOST IMPORTANT CHAKRAS. THEY ARE SIX CENTRES OF CONSCIOUSNESS WHICH ARE DISTRIBUTED INSIDE THE SPINAL COLUMN, AT THE BASE OF WHICH IS A LATENT ENERGY: **KUNDALINI**.

WHERE ARE THEY SITUATED?

AJNA: AT THE LEVEL OF THE PITUITARY GLAND. IT CONTROLS ALL THE OTHERS.

ANAHATA: AT THE LEVEL OF THE HEART.

VISHUDDHA: AT THE LEVEL OF THE THYROID.

SVADHISHTHANA: AT THE LEVEL OF THE SEX ORGANS.

MULADHARA: THE ROOT CHAKRA IS FOUND TWO FINGERS ABOVE THE ANUS.

AT THE TOP OF THE SKULL IS THE THOUSAND-PETALLED **LOTUS (SAHASRARA)**, THE SEAT OF ABSOLUTE CONSCIOUSNESS. THIS LOTUS BLOSSOMS WHEN THE YOGI ENTERS INTO SAMADHI.

MANIPURA: FOUR FINGERS BELOW THE NAVEL.

Chapter 5

PREPARING FOR POSTURES

Yoga is not just a series of physical jerks or gymnastics. Before you start the asanas, you should consider the first two limbs of yoga, which affect your mental attitude and are considered as a preparation for the postures. In turn the postures prepare the yoga student for deep mental concentration.

Yoga postures use all the joints of the body, but essentially they all involve the spinal column. They have several aims: to improve the function of organs inside the body; to ensure good blood circulation and a healthy, unobstructed nervous system, as well as aiding harmonious distribution of Prana and the removal of subconscious muscular tension.

Muscular tensions, originating in the mind, can cause organic disorders which lead to illness and disease. The East has never separated the physical from the psychological and discoveries about psychosomatic illness by Western doctors have shown the importance of this idea.

A place to practise

The best place to practise is a quiet room where you feel at ease. It should be airy, but not draughty. Make sure you have enough room to move in and spread a rug or mat on the floor for the sitting and lying postures.

Your clothes should be loose and unrestricting. Many people find that a leotard or swimming trunks (if it's warm enough) are ideal. You should be barefoot.

Try to do some yoga every day, for at least 15 to 20 minutes, longer if possible.

Before you start

Before you begin to follow the lessons, there are some points you should bear in mind.
1. The lessons in the book should take 10 to 12 weeks, if you work through them systematically.
2. Stay with each lesson until you know it thoroughly and feel comfortable with it. Each lesson is there to be enjoyed. Hurrying through defeats the object of doing yoga, as you cannot relax.
3. Work gradually with the postures, especially the difficult ones. If you persevere gently, you will be able to manage the ones that seemed impossible at the start.
4. The postures are arranged in a progressive order leading from the simple to the more advanced. You should follow this planned order. The lesson summary at the end of each lesson gives a full practice or short practices which can be alternated.
5. Don't force your body. Stop when discomfort becomes pain or when you feel strain in your face, eyes, ears or breathing. You're not in a competition and forcing postures only creates physical and mental tension.
6. Wait two hours after eating before starting postures and breathing exercises.
7. If you have heart trouble or are concerned about whether you should try particular postures, consult your doctor. Obviously if you have a bad back, you shouldn't try vigorous bending. If necessary, postures can be modified with the help of a yoga teacher.
8. During menstruation no strong abdominal movements or inverted poses should be tried.
9. The occasional relaxation periods between asanas are essential. You lie on your back or your stomach, or kneel for at least a minute. It may seem like a waste of time to you, but the relaxation periods allow the vibrations of the preceding asanas to die out before you start the next. You should always relax for a few seconds before starting the next asana.

33

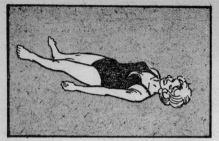

Relaxing on your back (Savasana)

Relaxing on your knees (Dharmikasana)

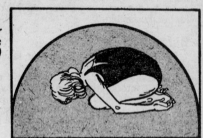

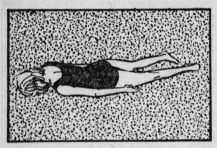

Relaxing on your front (Purvasana)

Melody and rhythm

A yoga session is considered a melody, where each asana is a note or chord which must be reached peacefully, in complete silence. Concentrate, don't speak. In time you will discover the benefits of silence and not find it difficult to perform the asanas without speaking.

Rhythm is also of great importance. Go into and out of asanas slowly, without hurrying your movements. Every posture performed on the right should be performed on the left in turn.

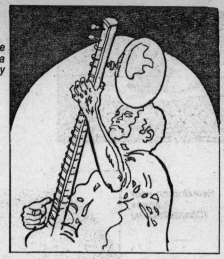

Imagine yoga as a melody

While holding the position, breathing should be normal, deep and through the nose, unless otherwise indicated.

A ballet

Every posture has one or more compensating counter-poses. A well-run session gives the impression to an onlooker of slow motion ballet where the dancers freeze into a series of graceful attitudes, flowing effortlessly from one posture to the next.

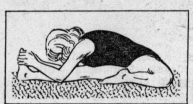

Posture: A forward bend

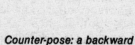

Counter-pose: a backward stretch

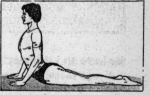

Concentration

When performing an asana, you must concentrate. Your undivided attention is essential, otherwise yoga asanas become a series of gymnastics. That may make you feel fit, but you will not be getting the full benefits that yoga can give you.

Chapter 6

LESSON ONE

Traditionally, the Guru (teacher) taught his Chela (pupil) by word of mouth. Concepts would be explained and discussed, systems tried out and philosophies memorised. Now in this book we shall be introducing new concepts with each of our five programmed lessons. Each concept is an idea to be explained and studied, but it has a practical application also, so it works on the mind and the body. For this first lesson the concept is being in a state of awareness of yourself.

Awareness breathing

Performed at the beginning of the lesson, this exercise turns the mind inward by closely observing how breathing works.

There are many financial or domestic distractions in life that draw your attention outward; and matters in the world at large which are beyond your control, to say nothing of your leisure and social activities. Even if you feel happy and contented generally, the plans and problems of daily life raise a serious barrier to the concentration you should be giving to the postures. If your thoughts are miles away, engaged in outside affairs, physical and psychological blocks form and obstruct the flow of energy that is created during a yoga session and you are losing some of its benefits.

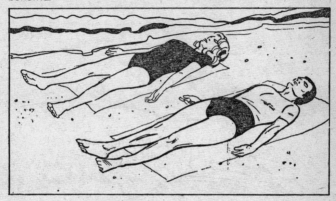

Relax and concentrate on your own breathing

The ideal is to free your mind from distractions and to centre it on yourself. Your mind should be calm and alert. Try to keep it focused throughout the practice. Listen to your own breathing which is stretched during the postures and the relaxation periods. You will find you return to the daily round later, physically and mentally refreshed.

Awareness standing

Tadasana (Mountain pose) is included at the beginning as it is concerned with standing correctly. We tend to take standing for granted until we stand about too long and develop aches and pains in our feet, legs or back. When you study the Mountain pose and find how good it feels to stand really well, you will understand how important this is. In fact the Mountain pose is the position in which many of the yoga movements start and finish.

Apart from making you look better, standing well gives the internal organs space and scope in which to function properly: the lungs inflate better, the heart and blood circulation operate at their best and the digestion is also helped along.

When you practise, you should think about the awareness concept also; yoga regards correct standing as another way of centring the mind and making it still.

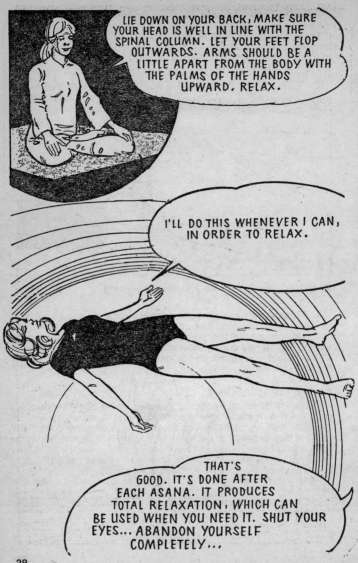

TADASANA - Mountain

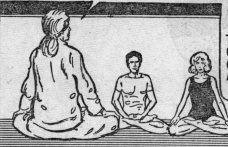

LEARN TO STAND CORRECTLY — THIS NEEDS SOME PRACTICE. THE STOMACH SHOULD BE IN BUT THE PELVIS SWAYS FORWARD A LITTLE. THE CHEST MUST BE OPEN, THE SHOULDERS SHOULDN'T BE HUNCHED. THE NAPE SHOULD BE STRETCHED UPWARD; DON'T POKE YOUR CHIN FORWARD. THE WEIGHT OF THE BODY SHOULD BE EQUALLY DISTRIBUTED OVER BOTH FEET, FROM TOES TO HEELS. THIS POSTURE CORRECTS THE MISSHAPING OF THE SPINAL COLUMN AND MAKES THE BODY MUSCULAR.

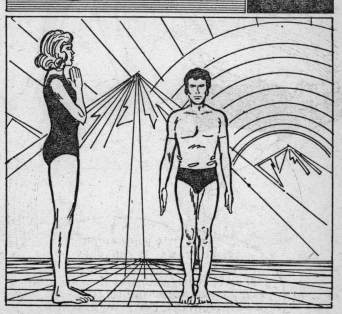

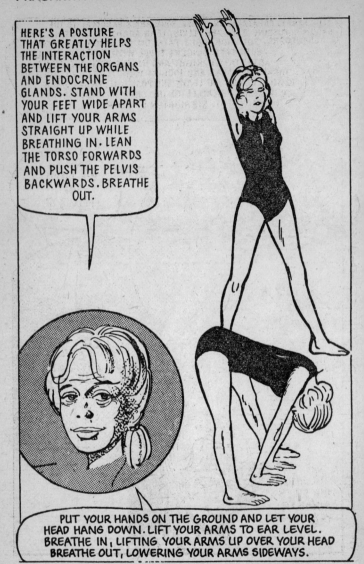

HERE'S A POSTURE THAT GREATLY HELPS THE INTERACTION BETWEEN THE ORGANS AND ENDOCRINE GLANDS. STAND WITH YOUR FEET WIDE APART AND LIFT YOUR ARMS STRAIGHT UP WHILE BREATHING IN. LEAN THE TORSO FORWARDS AND PUSH THE PELVIS BACKWARDS. BREATHE OUT.

PUT YOUR HANDS ON THE GROUND AND LET YOUR HEAD HANG DOWN. LIFT YOUR ARMS TO EAR LEVEL. BREATHE IN, LIFTING YOUR ARMS UP OVER YOUR HEAD BREATHE OUT, LOWERING YOUR ARMS SIDEWAYS.

TRIKONASANA — Triangles

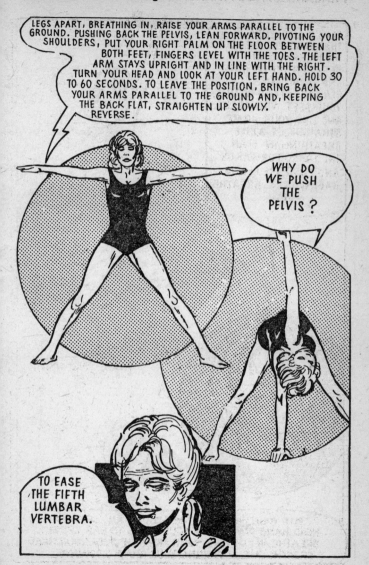

LEGS APART, BREATHING IN, RAISE YOUR ARMS PARALLEL TO THE GROUND. PUSHING BACK THE PELVIS, LEAN FORWARD. PIVOTING YOUR SHOULDERS, PUT YOUR RIGHT PALM ON THE FLOOR BETWEEN BOTH FEET, FINGERS LEVEL WITH THE TOES. THE LEFT ARM STAYS UPRIGHT AND IN LINE WITH THE RIGHT. TURN YOUR HEAD AND LOOK AT YOUR LEFT HAND. HOLD 30 TO 60 SECONDS. TO LEAVE THE POSITION, BRING BACK YOUR ARMS PARALLEL TO THE GROUND AND, KEEPING THE BACK FLAT, STRAIGHTEN UP SLOWLY. REVERSE.

WHY DO WE PUSH THE PELVIS?

TO EASE THE FIFTH LUMBAR VERTEBRA.

THIS IS A BASIC SITTING POSTURE, WHICH
IS COMFORTABLE FOR MEDITATION AND
BREATHING EXERCISES.
CROSS YOUR ANKLES AND PULL YOUR FEET
IN TOWARDS YOU. TRY TO KEEP YOUR
KNEES AS NEAR TO THE GROUND AS
POSSIBLE. KEEP YOUR BACK STRAIGHT,
WITH YOUR CHIN DOWN. REST YOUR
HANDS ON YOUR KNEES.
THE SUKHASANA WILL PREPARE YOU FOR
THE LOTUS POSTURE LATER ON.

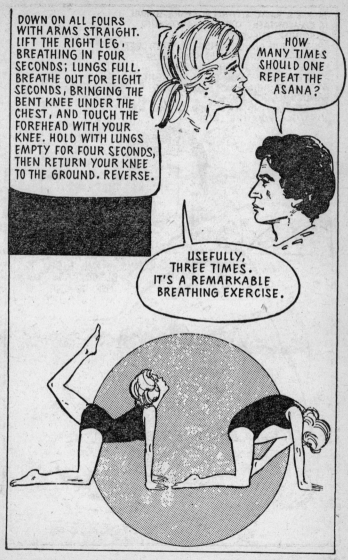

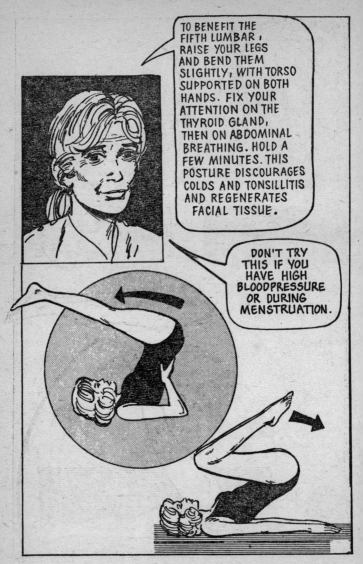

ARDHA SALABHASANA - Half Locust

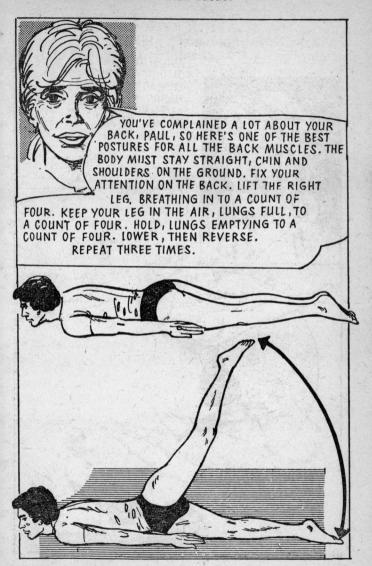

YOU'VE COMPLAINED A LOT ABOUT YOUR BACK, PAUL, SO HERE'S ONE OF THE BEST POSTURES FOR ALL THE BACK MUSCLES. THE BODY MUST STAY STRAIGHT, CHIN AND SHOULDERS ON THE GROUND. FIX YOUR ATTENTION ON THE BACK. LIFT THE RIGHT LEG, BREATHING IN TO A COUNT OF FOUR. KEEP YOUR LEG IN THE AIR, LUNGS FULL, TO A COUNT OF FOUR. HOLD, LUNGS EMPTYING TO A COUNT OF FOUR. LOWER, THEN REVERSE. REPEAT THREE TIMES.

ARMS EACH SIDE OF THE HEAD, BREATHE IN, RAISE LEGS AND BEND THEM. BREATHE OUT, LOWER THEM TO THE LEFT, TO THE FLOOR; TURN HEAD TO THE RIGHT. STAY LIKE THAT FOR A MINUTE, FIXING YOUR ATTENTION ON THE TORSION OF THE ABDOMEN. REPEAT OTHER SIDE.
VERY GOOD FOR THE ABDOMINAL ORGANS, LIVER, SPLEEN, AND PANCREAS.

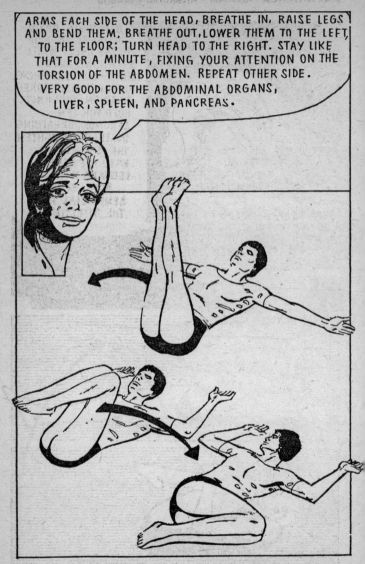

PAVANAMUKTASANA - Intestinal passage

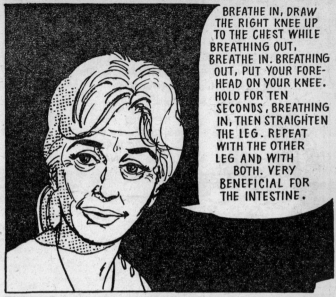

BREATHE IN, DRAW THE RIGHT KNEE UP TO THE CHEST WHILE BREATHING OUT, BREATHE IN. BREATHING OUT, PUT YOUR FOREHEAD ON YOUR KNEE. HOLD FOR TEN SECONDS, BREATHING IN, THEN STRAIGHTEN THE LEG. REPEAT WITH THE OTHER LEG AND WITH BOTH. VERY BENEFICIAL FOR THE INTESTINE.

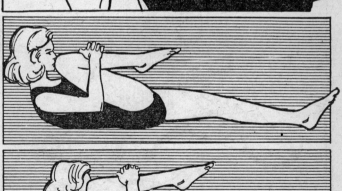

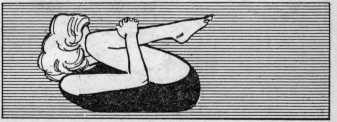

A bath of youth

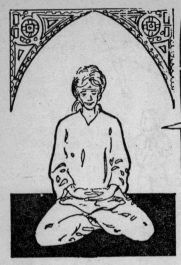

EACH TIME YOU PRACTISE OBSERVING THE RHYTHM PERFECTLY AND THE SEQUENCE OF ASANAS, YOU WILL HAVE CEASED TO FEEL ANY TIREDNESS. YOU WILL FEEL REFRESHED AND INVIGORATED AFTERWARDS.

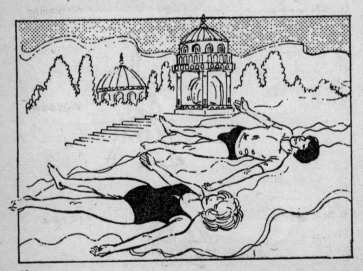

SUMMARY OF LESSON 1 FULL PRACTICE

1. Relaxation   2-5 mins

2. Awareness breathing   2-3 mins

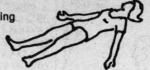

3. Mountain (static)   1-2 mins

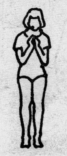

4. Feet apart   6-8 breaths

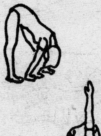

5. Triangles   30-60 secs

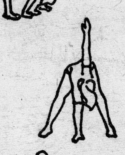

6. Easy pose   1-2 mins

49

7. Relaxation (on knees) 1-2 mins

8. Head on knees 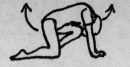 3 times each side

9. Reverse pose 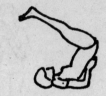 30-60 secs

10. Half locust 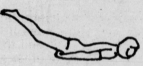 12 breaths on each leg. Repeat 3 times

11. Torsion of abdomen 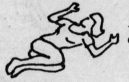 1 min each side

12. Intestinal passage 5 breaths each leg, then both legs together

13. Relaxation 1-3 mins

Key posture: Reverse pose
Short practice — Day A: postures 2, 4, 6, 8, 9, 10, 13
Short practice — Day B: postures 3, 5, 7, 8, 9, 11, 12, 13

Chapter 7

LESSON TWO

The new concept in this chapter is that each lesson has a key posture. In this case it is the Back half-stretched posture. You will find that this is also in both the short practices, together with the Cobra as a counterpose.

Vinyasa

The idea is that you work step by step up to the main asana. Then follows a posture to adjust or counter the effects of a particular move in one direction by a bend in the other direction. In this way the harmony of the body is maintained. Afterwards you gently come down again, usually through less strenuous exercises.

When you have worked on the various postures in a lesson and understand them, you will be able to look through each programme as a whole and you will see that it is planned according to this concept. The Sanskrit word for this is Vinyasa.

The earlier postures in a vinyasa are concerned with stretching and preparing the body through a whole series of asanas. This preparation usually means that when the main pose is reached it can be done more easily, held a little longer and performed without physical or mental strain. With normal precautions any risk of injury is eliminated. Then you work down from the main posture.

After your practice is completed it is likely that you will be going about your everyday business and making movements that include walking, sitting and carrying. The final postures are simpler and nearer to everyday activity to bring the bodily state back to normal.

The complete breath

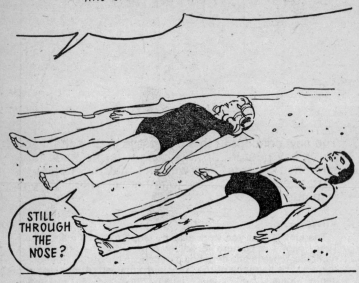

BRING YOUR ARMS DOWN BESIDE YOUR BODY, HANDS TURNED UPWARD. YOU ARE GOING TO COMBINE THE THREE KINDS OF BREATHING. START LOW WITH THE ABDOMEN, THEN THE MIDDLE OF THE CHEST, THEN THE TOP. SMOOTH AND SLOW. THAT'S RIGHT.

STILL THROUGH THE NOSE?

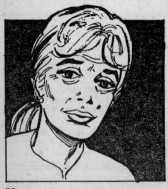

YES OPEN THE NOSTRILS, BUT CONTRACT THE PHARYNX SLIGHTLY AND LET YOUR TONGUE LIE LIMP, OR COME UP A BIT OVER THE UPPER TEETH.

TADASANA — Mountain dynamic

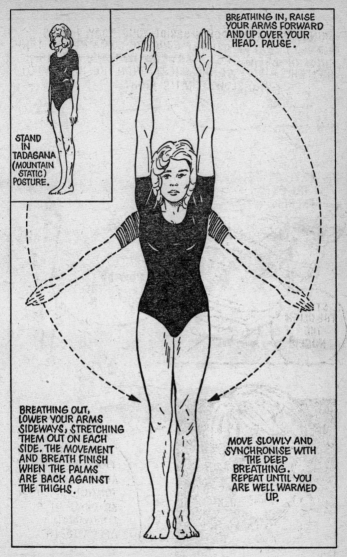

STAND IN TADASANA (MOUNTAIN STATIC) POSTURE.

BREATHING IN, RAISE YOUR ARMS FORWARD AND UP OVER YOUR HEAD. PAUSE.

BREATHING OUT, LOWER YOUR ARMS SIDEWAYS, STRETCHING THEM OUT ON EACH SIDE. THE MOVEMENT AND BREATH FINISH WHEN THE PALMS ARE BACK AGAINST THE THIGHS.

MOVE SLOWLY AND SYNCHRONISE WITH THE DEEP BREATHING. REPEAT UNTIL YOU ARE WELL WARMED UP.

PADANGUSTHASANA - Big toes

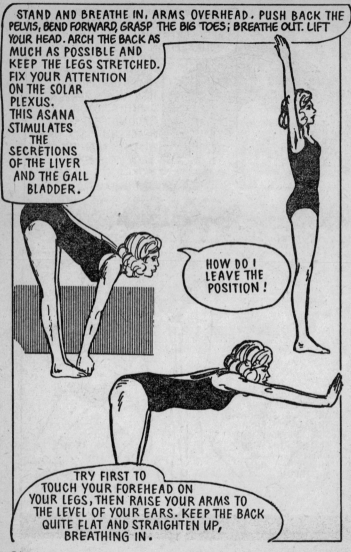

STAND AND BREATHE IN, ARMS OVERHEAD. PUSH BACK THE PELVIS, BEND FORWARD, GRASP THE BIG TOES; BREATHE OUT. LIFT YOUR HEAD. ARCH THE BACK AS MUCH AS POSSIBLE AND KEEP THE LEGS STRETCHED. FIX YOUR ATTENTION ON THE SOLAR PLEXUS. THIS ASANA STIMULATES THE SECRETIONS OF THE LIVER AND THE GALL BLADDER.

HOW DO I LEAVE THE POSITION!

TRY FIRST TO TOUCH YOUR FOREHEAD ON YOUR LEGS, THEN RAISE YOUR ARMS TO THE LEVEL OF YOUR EARS. KEEP THE BACK QUITE FLAT AND STRAIGHTEN UP, BREATHING IN.

MANDUKASANA - Standing frog

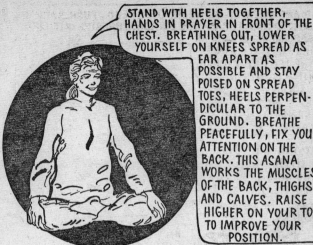

STAND WITH HEELS TOGETHER, HANDS IN PRAYER IN FRONT OF THE CHEST. BREATHING OUT, LOWER YOURSELF ON KNEES SPREAD AS FAR APART AS POSSIBLE AND STAY POISED ON SPREAD TOES, HEELS PERPENDICULAR TO THE GROUND. BREATHE PEACEFULLY, FIX YOUR ATTENTION ON THE BACK. THIS ASANA WORKS THE MUSCLES OF THE BACK, THIGHS, AND CALVES. RAISE HIGHER ON YOUR TOES TO IMPROVE YOUR POSITION.

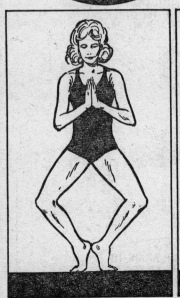

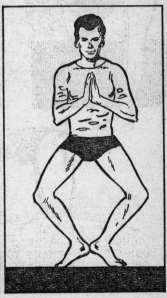

VRIKSHASANA - Tree

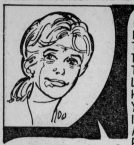

STAND WELL BALANCED, LIFT ONE FOOT AND PUT IT ACROSS THE OTHER THIGH AS IN THE LOTUS. STRETCH THE ARMS OUT IN FRONT, LETTING THE HANDS HANG LOOSELY. OPEN YOUR ARMS, BREATHING IN, AND STRETCH THEM ABOVE YOUR HEAD, PRESSING THE PALMS TOGETHER. HOLD FOR A FEW SECONDS, BREATHING DEEPLY, WITH YOUR ATTENTION ON THE AJNA CHAKRA. ON COMING OUT OF THE POSTURE THE HANDS ARE BROUGHT BACK IN FRONT OF THE CHEST IN PRAYER. REVERSE.

PAUL, AS YOU CAN'T GET YOUR FOOT INTO THE LOTUS PUT THE SOLE ON THE INSIDE OF THE OTHER THIGH. KEEP THE THIGH-BONE PARALLEL TO THE FLOOR.

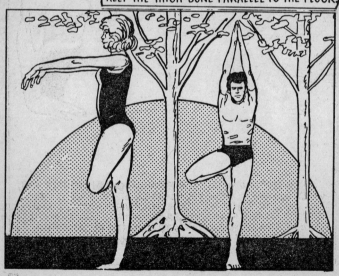

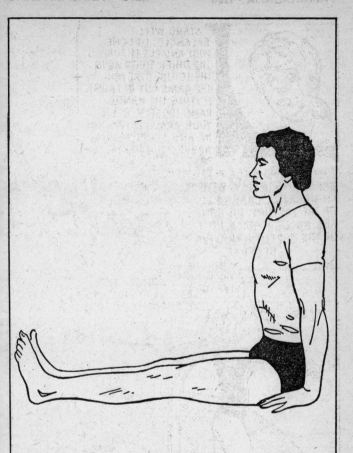

SIT ON THE FLOOR WITH THE LEGS STRAIGHT OUT IN FRONT OF YOU, THEN SIT FORWARD ON THE PELVIC BONES, SO THE BASE OF THE SPINE DOES NOT TOUCH THE FLOOR. PUSH YOUR HANDS DOWN ON THE FLOOR TO HELP KEEP YOUR BACK UPRIGHT AND YOUR CHEST FORWARD. IF YOUR BACK STARTS TO ACHE, IT'S BECAUSE THE MUSCLES ARE STILL WEAK. PRACTISING WITH YOUR BACK AGAINST THE WALL WILL HELP.

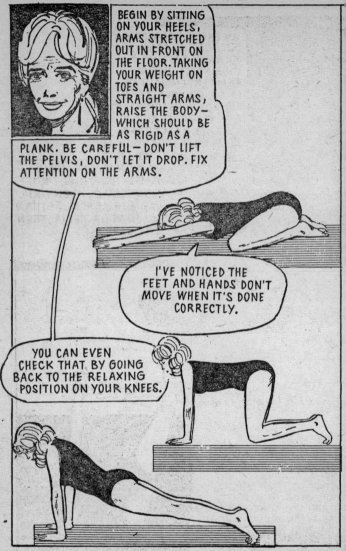

BEGIN BY SITTING ON YOUR HEELS, ARMS STRETCHED OUT IN FRONT ON THE FLOOR. TAKING YOUR WEIGHT ON TOES AND STRAIGHT ARMS, RAISE THE BODY— WHICH SHOULD BE AS RIGID AS A PLANK. BE CAREFUL— DON'T LIFT THE PELVIS, DON'T LET IT DROP. FIX ATTENTION ON THE ARMS.

I'VE NOTICED THE FEET AND HANDS DON'T MOVE WHEN IT'S DONE CORRECTLY.

YOU CAN EVEN CHECK THAT BY GOING BACK TO THE RELAXING POSITION ON YOUR KNEES.

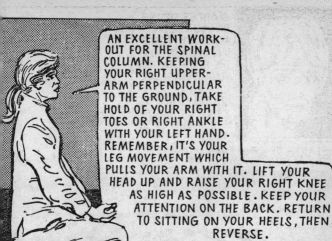

AN EXCELLENT WORK-OUT FOR THE SPINAL COLUMN. KEEPING YOUR RIGHT UPPER-ARM PERPENDICULAR TO THE GROUND, TAKE HOLD OF YOUR RIGHT TOES OR RIGHT ANKLE WITH YOUR LEFT HAND. REMEMBER, IT'S YOUR LEG MOVEMENT WHICH PULLS YOUR ARM WITH IT. LIFT YOUR HEAD UP AND RAISE YOUR RIGHT KNEE AS HIGH AS POSSIBLE. KEEP YOUR ATTENTION ON THE BACK. RETURN TO SITTING ON YOUR HEELS, THEN REVERSE.

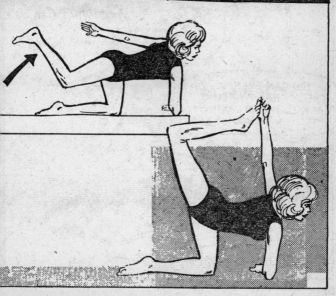

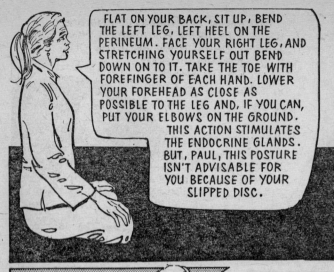

FLAT ON YOUR BACK, SIT UP, BEND THE LEFT LEG, LEFT HEEL ON THE PERINEUM. FACE YOUR RIGHT LEG, AND STRETCHING YOURSELF OUT BEND DOWN ON TO IT. TAKE THE TOE WITH FOREFINGER OF EACH HAND. LOWER YOUR FOREHEAD AS CLOSE AS POSSIBLE TO THE LEG AND, IF YOU CAN, PUT YOUR ELBOWS ON THE GROUND. THIS ACTION STIMULATES THE ENDOCRINE GLANDS. BUT, PAUL, THIS POSTURE ISN'T ADVISABLE FOR YOU BECAUSE OF YOUR SLIPPED DISC.

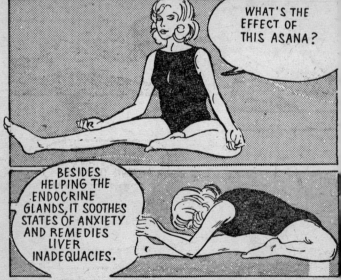

WHAT'S THE EFFECT OF THIS ASANA?

BESIDES HELPING THE ENDOCRINE GLANDS, IT SOOTHES STATES OF ANXIETY AND REMEDIES LIVER INADEQUACIES.

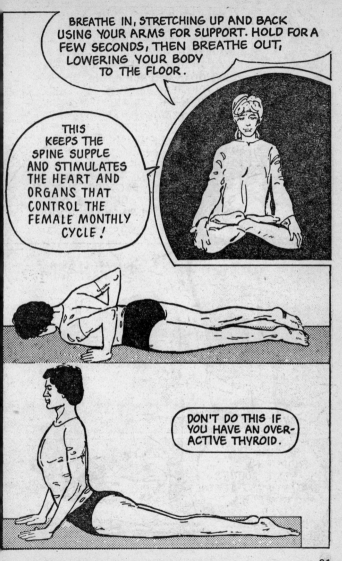

BREATHE IN, STRETCHING UP AND BACK USING YOUR ARMS FOR SUPPORT. HOLD FOR A FEW SECONDS, THEN BREATHE OUT, LOWERING YOUR BODY TO THE FLOOR.

THIS KEEPS THE SPINE SUPPLE AND STIMULATES THE HEART AND ORGANS THAT CONTROL THE FEMALE MONTHLY CYCLE!

DON'T DO THIS IF YOU HAVE AN OVER-ACTIVE THYROID.

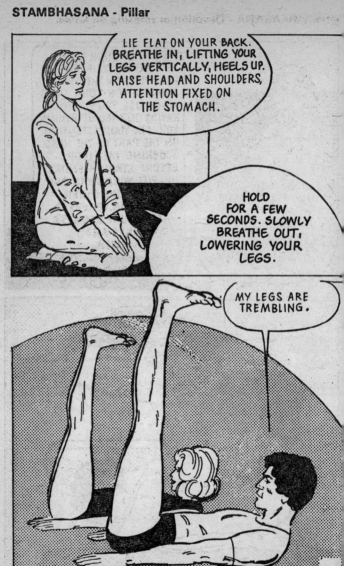

DHARMIKASANA - Devotion or relaxing on knees

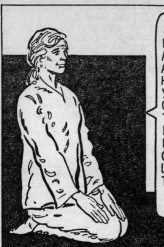

START ON YOUR KNEES, SITTING ON YOUR HEELS FOREHEAD ON THE GROUND, AND POSITION YOUR ARMS ALONGSIDE YOUR BODY, HANDS TURNED UP BEHIND YOU. FIX YOUR ATTENTION ON THE PART OF THE HEAD TOUCHING THE FLOOR. BEFORE STRAIGHTENING UP, PUT YOUR FISTS ONE ON TOP OF THE OTHER UNDER YOUR FOREHEAD. THIS POSTURE RELIEVES HEADACHES AND NAUSEA.

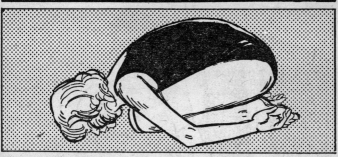

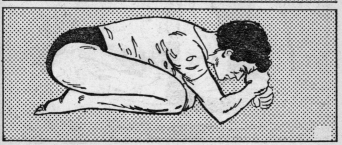

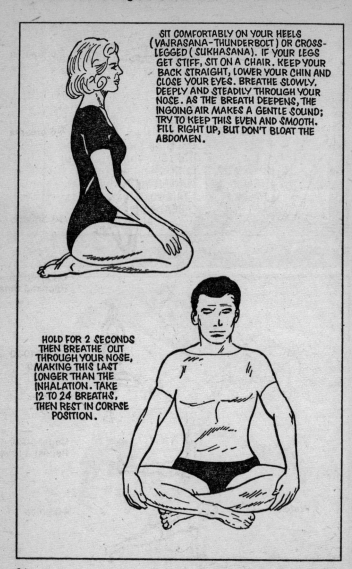

SIT COMFORTABLY ON YOUR HEELS (VAJRASANA-THUNDERBOLT) OR CROSS-LEGGED (SUKHASANA). IF YOUR LEGS GET STIFF, SIT ON A CHAIR. KEEP YOUR BACK STRAIGHT, LOWER YOUR CHIN AND CLOSE YOUR EYES. BREATHE SLOWLY, DEEPLY AND STEADILY THROUGH YOUR NOSE. AS THE BREATH DEEPENS, THE INGOING AIR MAKES A GENTLE SOUND; TRY TO KEEP THIS EVEN AND SMOOTH. FILL RIGHT UP, BUT DON'T BLOAT THE ABDOMEN.

HOLD FOR 2 SECONDS THEN BREATHE OUT THROUGH YOUR NOSE, MAKING THIS LAST LONGER THAN THE INHALATION. TAKE 12 TO 24 BREATHS, THEN REST IN CORPSE POSITION.

SUMMARY OF LESSON 2 FULL PRACTICE

1. Relaxation — 2-5 mins

2. Complete breath — 6-8 breaths

3. Mountain (dynamic) — 6-8 breaths

4. Big toes — 6-8 breaths

5. Standing frog — Count to 20. Repeat 3 times

6. Tree — Count 10-20 each leg

7. Relaxation — 1-2 mins

8. Staff — Count 10-20. Repeat 3 times

9. Watcher — 4-6 holds

10. Half arch 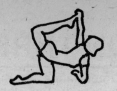 3 times
each side

11. Back half-stretched 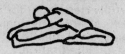 3 times
each side

12. Cobra 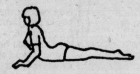 Count 5-10.
Repeat 3 times

13. Pillar 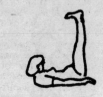 10-12 times

14. Devotion 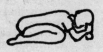 12 slow
breaths

15. Ujjayi breathing 12-24 breaths

16. Relaxation 2-3 mins

Key posture: Back half-stretched
Short practice — Day A: postures 3, 5, 7, 8, 10, 11, 12, 15, 16
Short practice — Day B: postures 4, 6, 7, 9, 10, 11, 12, 13, 14

Chapter 8

LESSON THREE

In yoga great importance is attached to breathing and it is this aspect that lesson three covers. Good breathing helps people in good health, and can prove wonderfully beneficial for the person who can only do a few of the physical exercises, due to incapacity, age or ill health. It is also an aid to concentration and meditation.

Pranayama

The Sanskrit name comprises two words which mean life force and control. It is the fourth in the Eight Limbs of Yoga.

Life force comes from food, sunshine, sleep, water and air. The vital factor is air, and your aim in the first few weeks should be the straightforward and basic one of improving your normal breathing. This is best done by working for short periods on Ujjayi, as described in lesson two. It can be practised at odd moments when sitting upright in a chair or when out walking. Do not go beyond what is comfortable with breathing. Keep alert and sensitive to ensure that there is never any strain; your facial muscles and shoulders, should not become tense.

Quite unconsciously, many people breathe too rapidly and too shallowly. Over the years this means an inadequate intake of oxygen and a reduced supply of Prana (life force). Shallow breathing also makes it harder for the lungs to discharge fully the waste matter produced in the respiratory process.

With slightly deeper normal breathing everything works better and the condition and functions of the blood improve. The diaphragm will develop a better action with consequent benefits to the internal organs and the digestion.

A breathing exercise has been included in each of the five lessons so that gradually, with careful attention, you may develop this function by learning to control the breath and master its uses. In time it will prove a means of generally raising your overall state of health.

There is also a psychological aspect to breathing, when the mental condition is reflected in the way a person breathes. Compare your breathing when you're nervous or excited with the slow rhythm when you are relaxed and calm. Think of how you glow with confidence and optimism when you've been out for a walk and taken a good breath of fresh air.

Finally, yoga considers breathing to be a link between body and mind, between the conscious and the subconscious mind. Breathing is regarded as a pathway along which you travel from outer activities, such as behaviour and asanas, to inner activities, such as concentration and meditation. It focuses the attention and stills the mind.

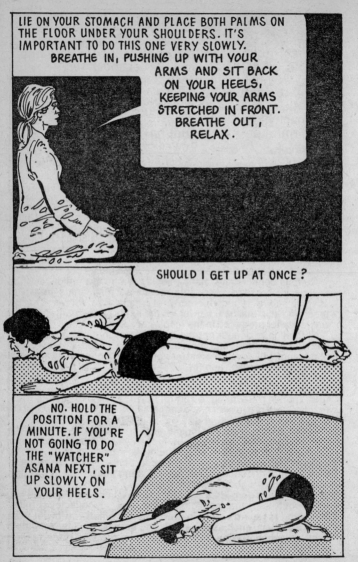

LIE ON YOUR STOMACH AND PLACE BOTH PALMS ON THE FLOOR UNDER YOUR SHOULDERS. IT'S IMPORTANT TO DO THIS ONE VERY SLOWLY. BREATHE IN, PUSHING UP WITH YOUR ARMS AND SIT BACK ON YOUR HEELS, KEEPING YOUR ARMS STRETCHED IN FRONT. BREATHE OUT, RELAX.

SHOULD I GET UP AT ONCE?

NO. HOLD THE POSITION FOR A MINUTE. IF YOU'RE NOT GOING TO DO THE "WATCHER" ASANA NEXT, SIT UP SLOWLY ON YOUR HEELS.

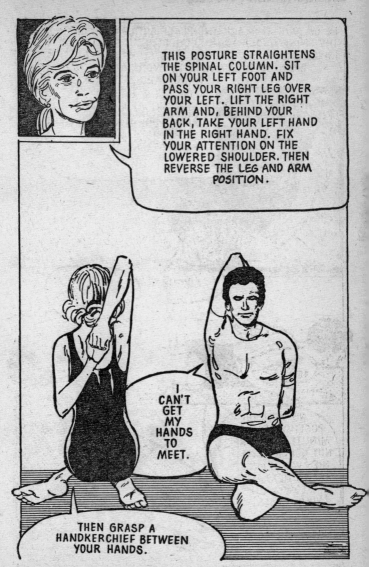

THIS POSTURE STRAIGHTENS THE SPINAL COLUMN. SIT ON YOUR LEFT FOOT AND PASS YOUR RIGHT LEG OVER YOUR LEFT. LIFT THE RIGHT ARM AND, BEHIND YOUR BACK, TAKE YOUR LEFT HAND IN THE RIGHT HAND. FIX YOUR ATTENTION ON THE LOWERED SHOULDER. THEN REVERSE THE LEG AND ARM POSITION.

I CAN'T GET MY HANDS TO MEET.

THEN GRASP A HANDKERCHIEF BETWEEN YOUR HANDS.

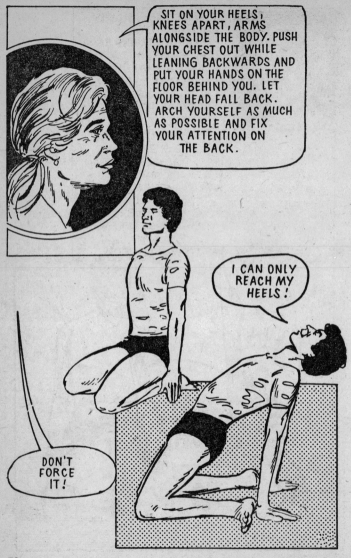

SARVANGASANA - Shoulder-stand or candle

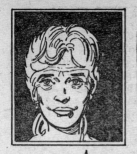

ON THE BACK, SLOWLY LIFT YOUR LEGS STRAIGHT UP AND RAISE THE PELVIS. BUT IF YOU CAN'T MANAGE IT, BEND YOUR LEGS TO BEGIN WITH. THE BODY SHOULD BE STRAIGHT AND BALANCED ON THE NAPE AND SHOULDERS, THE HANDS SUPPORTING THE BACK ABOVE THE KIDNEYS. ATTENTION IS FIXED ON THE THYROID GLAND. WHEN YOU CAN BALANCE PERFECTLY, HOLD THE POSITION FOR THREE MINUTES. IT'S IDEAL FOR EASING THE LEGS AFTER LONG STANDING. RELAX IN CORPSE POSITION FOR 1-2 MINS.
DON'T DO THIS DURING MENSTRUATION

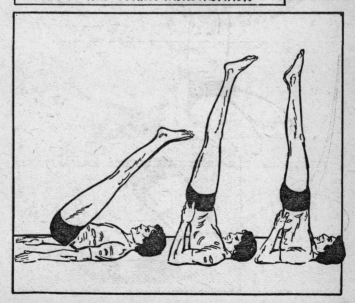

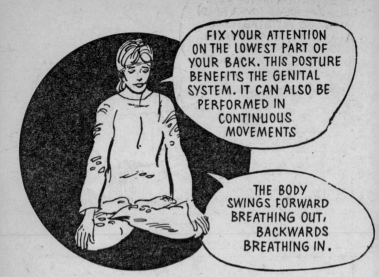

FIX YOUR ATTENTION ON THE LOWEST PART OF YOUR BACK. THIS POSTURE BENEFITS THE GENITAL SYSTEM. IT CAN ALSO BE PERFORMED IN CONTINUOUS MOVEMENTS

THE BODY SWINGS FORWARD BREATHING OUT, BACKWARDS BREATHING IN.

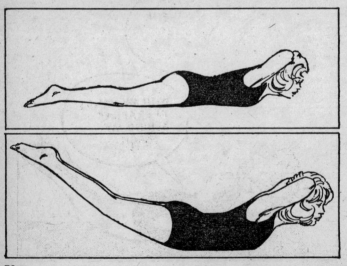

NAUKASANA - Boat

FIX ATTENTION ON THE BACK. LIE WITH ARMS (OVER HEAD) AND LEGS OUTSTRETCHED. BREATHE IN, RAISING ARMS, HEAD AND LEGS FROM THE FLOOR. HOLD, BREATHE OUT AND RELAX.

I LIKE TO DO IT WITH ARMS AND LEGS APART AND STRETCHED.

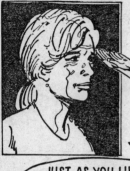

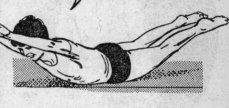

JUST AS YOU LIKE. PAUL, YOU LIKE THE DYNAMIC POSTURE, YOU CAN SWING TO THE RHYTHM OF YOUR BREATHING. JENNY LIKES THE STATIC POSITION.

...WITH MY HANDS "IN PRAYER" BEHIND MY BACK.

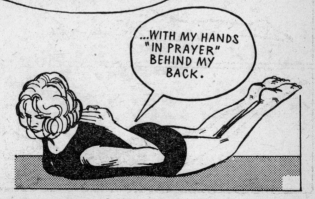

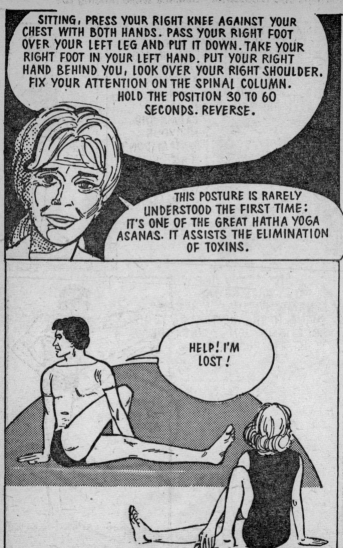

SITTING, PRESS YOUR RIGHT KNEE AGAINST YOUR CHEST WITH BOTH HANDS. PASS YOUR RIGHT FOOT OVER YOUR LEFT LEG AND PUT IT DOWN. TAKE YOUR RIGHT FOOT IN YOUR LEFT HAND. PUT YOUR RIGHT HAND BEHIND YOU, LOOK OVER YOUR RIGHT SHOULDER. FIX YOUR ATTENTION ON THE SPINAL COLUMN. HOLD THE POSITION 30 TO 60 SECONDS. REVERSE.

THIS POSTURE IS RARELY UNDERSTOOD THE FIRST TIME; IT'S ONE OF THE GREAT HATHA YOGA ASANAS. IT ASSISTS THE ELIMINATION OF TOXINS.

HELP! I'M LOST!

PADANGUSTHASANA - Balance while holding toe

STANDING, LIFT YOUR RIGHT LEG TOWARDS YOUR CHEST UNTIL YOU CAN TAKE THE TOE IN YOUR RIGHT HAND. STRETCH THE LEG OUT IN FRONT OF YOU AND PUT YOUR LEFT HAND ON YOUR HIP. FIX YOUR ATTENTION ON THE AJNA CHAKRA BETWEEN THE BROWS. THE ASANA CALMS THE NERVOUS SYSTEM. DON'T LEAN OVER, PAUL, YOU'LL LOSE YOUR BALANCE.

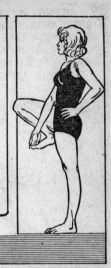

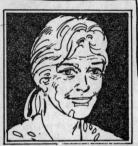

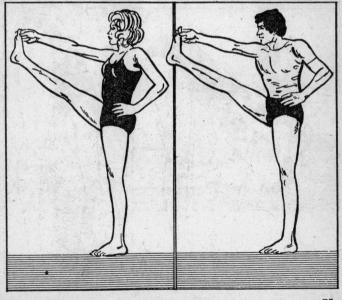

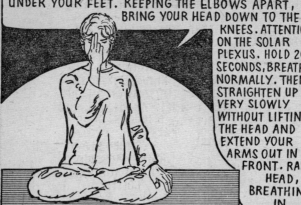

THIS ASANA SLIMS THE STOMACH AND HIPS, BUT IT'S NOT FOR YOU, PAUL, WITH YOUR SLIPPED DISC. STAND LEGS SLIGHTLY APART, BEND AND SLIDE YOUR HANDS UNDER YOUR FEET. KEEPING THE ELBOWS APART, BRING YOUR HEAD DOWN TO THE KNEES. ATTENTION ON THE SOLAR PLEXUS. HOLD 20 SECONDS, BREATHING NORMALLY. THEN STRAIGHTEN UP VERY SLOWLY WITHOUT LIFTING THE HEAD AND EXTEND YOUR ARMS OUT IN FRONT. RAISE HEAD, BREATHING IN.

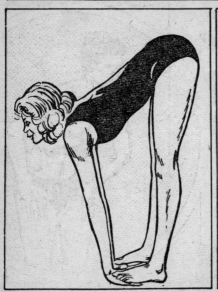

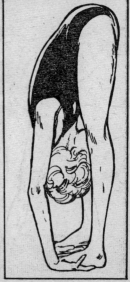

UDDIYANA BHANDAA — Flying contraction

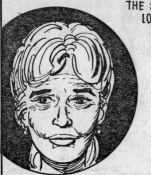

THIS CONTRACTION HELPS THE CIRCULATION OF PRANA AND THE ABDOMINAL ENERGY. BEND KNEES SLIGHTLY, HANDS ON THIGHS, CHIN LOWERED TOWARD THE CHEST, AND BREATHE IN DEEPLY. EXHALE COMPLETELY TO BRING THE STOMACH UP TO THE LOWER PART OF THE THORAX, AND PRESS THE HANDS ON THE THIGHS. FIX YOUR ATTENTION ON THE SOLAR PLEXUS. HOLD 5 TO 10 SECONDS BREATHE SEVERAL TIMES THEN REPEAT THREE TIMES. DON'T DO THIS IF YOU HAVE COLITIS.

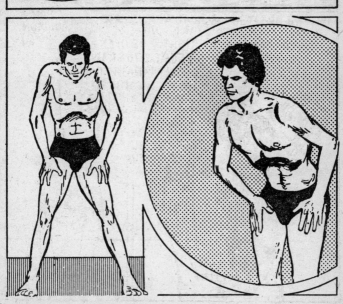

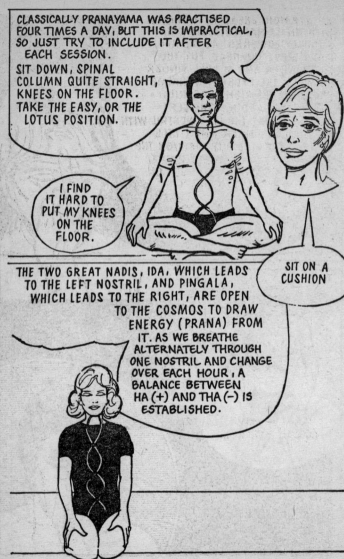

CLASSICALLY PRANAYAMA WAS PRACTISED FOUR TIMES A DAY, BUT THIS IS IMPRACTICAL, SO JUST TRY TO INCLUDE IT AFTER EACH SESSION.

SIT DOWN, SPINAL COLUMN QUITE STRAIGHT, KNEES ON THE FLOOR. TAKE THE EASY, OR THE LOTUS POSITION.

I FIND IT HARD TO PUT MY KNEES ON THE FLOOR.

THE TWO GREAT NADIS, IDA, WHICH LEADS TO THE LEFT NOSTRIL, AND PINGALA, WHICH LEADS TO THE RIGHT, ARE OPEN TO THE COSMOS TO DRAW ENERGY (PRANA) FROM IT. AS WE BREATHE ALTERNATELY THROUGH ONE NOSTRIL AND CHANGE OVER EACH HOUR, A BALANCE BETWEEN HA (+) AND THA (−) IS ESTABLISHED.

SIT ON A CUSHION

Breathing to clear the Nadis

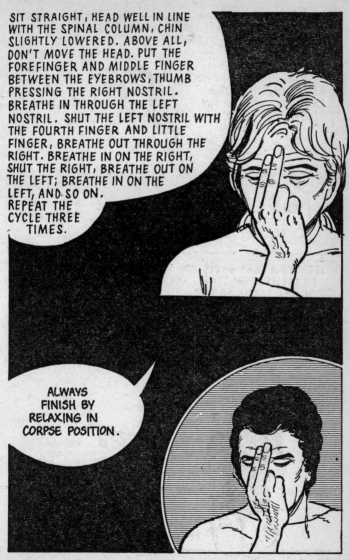

SIT STRAIGHT, HEAD WELL IN LINE WITH THE SPINAL COLUMN, CHIN SLIGHTLY LOWERED. ABOVE ALL, DON'T MOVE THE HEAD. PUT THE FOREFINGER AND MIDDLE FINGER BETWEEN THE EYEBROWS, THUMB PRESSING THE RIGHT NOSTRIL. BREATHE IN THROUGH THE LEFT NOSTRIL. SHUT THE LEFT NOSTRIL WITH THE FOURTH FINGER AND LITTLE FINGER, BREATHE OUT THROUGH THE RIGHT. BREATHE IN ON THE RIGHT, SHUT THE RIGHT, BREATHE OUT ON THE LEFT; BREATHE IN ON THE LEFT, AND SO ON. REPEAT THE CYCLE THREE TIMES.

ALWAYS FINISH BY RELAXING IN CORPSE POSITION.

SUMMARY OF LESSON 3 FULL PRACTICE

1. The adept 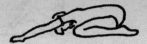 Count 40-60 slowly

2. Cow's head Count 30-60 each arm

3. Kneeling frog 5-10 breaths. Repeat 3 times

4. Shoulder stand 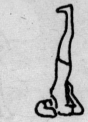 1-3 mins

5. Relaxation 1-2 mins

6. Crocodile 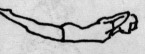 4-6 holds, relax front down in between: if swinging 6 breaths

7. Boat 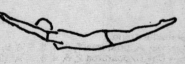 3-6 holds, relax front down in between: if swinging 6 breaths

8. Twisting　　　　　　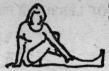　　　Count 30-60
each side

9. Relaxation (on knees)　　　　　2-5 mins

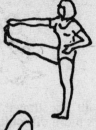

10. Balance　　　　　　　　　Count 5-10
each leg

11. Stork　　　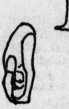　　　Count 20.
Repeat 3 times

12. Flying contraction　　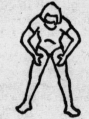　　Hold 5-10 secs.
Repeat 3 times

13. Relaxation　　　　　　　　1-2 mins

14. Alternate nostril　　　　Count 5-8 for
breathing in/out.
Repeat 3-8 times

15. Relaxation　　　　　　　　1-2 mins

Key posture: Shoulder stand
Short practice — Day A: postures 1, 3, 4, 5, 6, 8, 9, 11, 14, 15
Short practice — Day B: postures 2, 3, 4, 5, 7, 9, 10, 12, 15

Chapter 9

LESSON FOUR

Many people will find that the postures in lessons four and five are more difficult. Not only will some of them be more difficult to get into and hold, but they are likely to demand more of your strength, suppleness, control and balance. It will become interesting for you to notice how, by now, you have become quite adept at many asanas in the earlier lessons. But you will feel like a beginner when you start work on some of these later ones. It is quite normal to be operating at different levels in this way in yoga.

Treat postures with respect

Remember postures at all stages of progress must be treated with respect. They are all more rigorous than is at first realised, and at times it is essential to work very carefully. The mind must be sensitive and alert to what you are doing.

In yoga you're not competing against others or against yourself. The effort, attitude and degree of concentration are what matters. All these are more important than any particular end result in the physical sense. Bear in mind the idea of yoga as a ballet and a melody.

Stirra and Sukha

The first word means firmness, stability; the second, comfort and lack of tension. These qualities may seem opposed, but in yoga they are extremely compatible. In fact, you should seek firmness with relaxation in each of the postures you work on. When you are in a particular hold, fix your attention on these two qualities and on the feel of the posture and how you are holding it. This is why you must work within your capacity and not strain yourself.

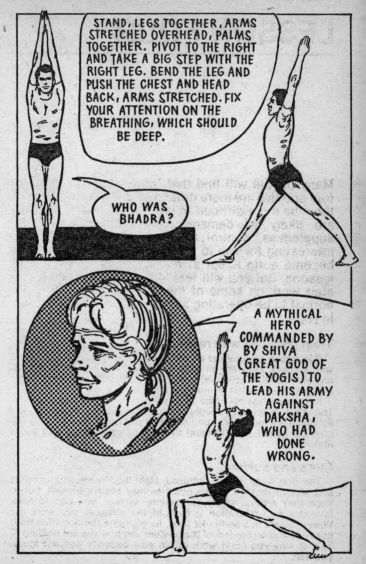

STAND, LEGS TOGETHER, ARMS STRETCHED OVERHEAD, PALMS TOGETHER. PIVOT TO THE RIGHT AND TAKE A BIG STEP WITH THE RIGHT LEG. BEND THE LEG AND PUSH THE CHEST AND HEAD BACK, ARMS STRETCHED. FIX YOUR ATTENTION ON THE BREATHING, WHICH SHOULD BE DEEP.

WHO WAS BHADRA?

A MYTHICAL HERO COMMANDED BY BY SHIVA (GREAT GOD OF THE YOGIS) TO LEAD HIS ARMY AGAINST DAKSHA, WHO HAD DONE WRONG.

UTTHITA TRIKONASANA - Stretched triangle

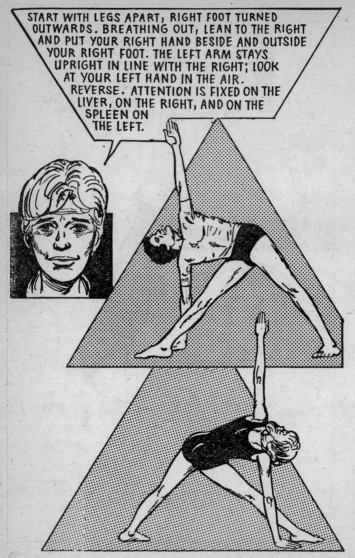

START WITH LEGS APART, RIGHT FOOT TURNED OUTWARDS. BREATHING OUT, LEAN TO THE RIGHT AND PUT YOUR RIGHT HAND BESIDE AND OUTSIDE YOUR RIGHT FOOT. THE LEFT ARM STAYS UPRIGHT IN LINE WITH THE RIGHT; LOOK AT YOUR LEFT HAND IN THE AIR. REVERSE. ATTENTION IS FIXED ON THE LIVER, ON THE RIGHT, AND ON THE SPLEEN ON THE LEFT.

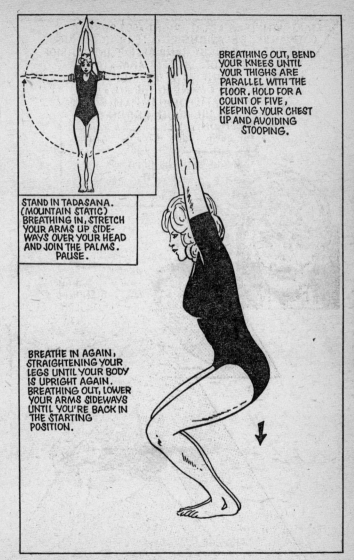

STAND IN TADASANA. (MOUNTAIN STATIC) BREATHING IN, STRETCH YOUR ARMS UP SIDEWAYS OVER YOUR HEAD AND JOIN THE PALMS. PAUSE.

BREATHING OUT, BEND YOUR KNEES UNTIL YOUR THIGHS ARE PARALLEL WITH THE FLOOR. HOLD FOR A COUNT OF FIVE, KEEPING YOUR CHEST UP AND AVOIDING STOOPING.

BREATHE IN AGAIN, STRAIGHTENING YOUR LEGS UNTIL YOUR BODY IS UPRIGHT AGAIN. BREATHING OUT, LOWER YOUR ARMS SIDEWAYS UNTIL YOU'RE BACK IN THE STARTING POSITION.

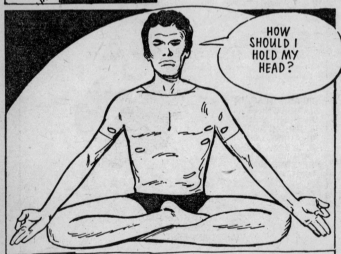

WE SHOULD ALL KNOW HOW TO DO THIS MEDITATION ASANA. THE LEFT HEEL IS DRAWN UNDER THE PERINEUM, THE TOES OF THE RIGHT FOOT ARE INSERTED BETWEEN THE CALF AND THE LEFT THIGH. PLACE THE BACK OF YOUR HANDS ON YOUR KNEES IN JNANA MUDRA, THE FOREFINGER TOUCHING THE TOP OF THE THUMB, THE OTHER FINGERS STRETCHED OUT. THE SPINE IS HELD STRAIGHT.

HOW SHOULD I HOLD MY HEAD?

STRETCH THE NAPE UPWARD AND LOWER THE CHIN A LITTLE TOWARD THE CHEST. FIX YOUR ATTENTION ON THE AJNA CHAKRA BETWEEN THE EYEBROWS.

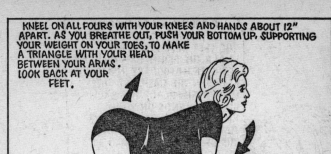

KNEEL ON ALL FOURS WITH YOUR KNEES AND HANDS ABOUT 12" APART. AS YOU BREATHE OUT, PUSH YOUR BOTTOM UP, SUPPORTING YOUR WEIGHT ON YOUR TOES, TO MAKE A TRIANGLE WITH YOUR HEAD BETWEEN YOUR ARMS. LOOK BACK AT YOUR FEET.

GENTLY TRY LOWERING YOUR HEELS TOWARDS THE FLOOR, STRETCHING THE HAMSTRINGS. HOLD THIS FOR A COUNT OF 6-10 BREATHING NORMALLY. COME BACK ON TO ALL FOURS, PAUSE AND REPEAT.

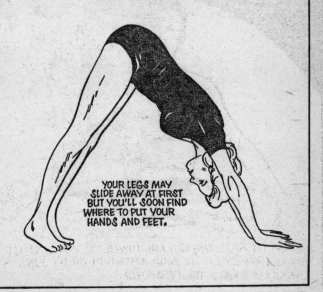

YOUR LEGS MAY SLIDE AWAY AT FIRST BUT YOU'LL SOON FIND WHERE TO PUT YOUR HANDS AND FEET.

PASHIMOTTANASANA - Stretching the West (back) of the body

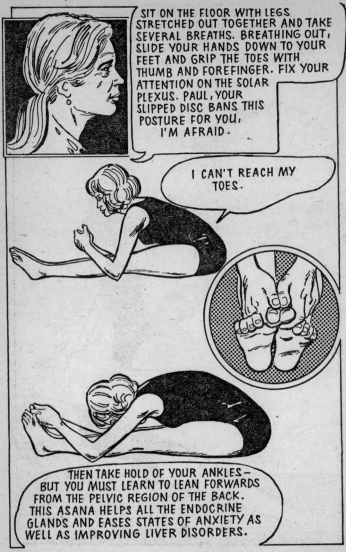

SIT ON THE FLOOR WITH LEGS STRETCHED OUT TOGETHER AND TAKE SEVERAL BREATHS. BREATHING OUT, SLIDE YOUR HANDS DOWN TO YOUR FEET AND GRIP THE TOES WITH THUMB AND FOREFINGER. FIX YOUR ATTENTION ON THE SOLAR PLEXUS. PAUL, YOUR SLIPPED DISC BANS THIS POSTURE FOR YOU, I'M AFRAID.

I CAN'T REACH MY TOES.

THEN TAKE HOLD OF YOUR ANKLES — BUT YOU MUST LEARN TO LEAN FORWARDS FROM THE PELVIC REGION OF THE BACK. THIS ASANA HELPS ALL THE ENDOCRINE GLANDS AND EASES STATES OF ANXIETY AS WELL AS IMPROVING LIVER DISORDERS.

PURVOTTANASANA - Stretching the East (front) of the body

STRETCHING THE EAST (FRONT) OF THE BODY. SIT AND LEAN BACK. RAISE YOUR BODY, KEEPING IT QUITE STRAIGHT, WITH FEET FLAT ON THE GROUND, HEAD FALLING BACK. FIX YOUR ATTENTION ON THE ARMS. THIS POSTURE STRENGTHENS THE ARMS AND SHOULDERS.

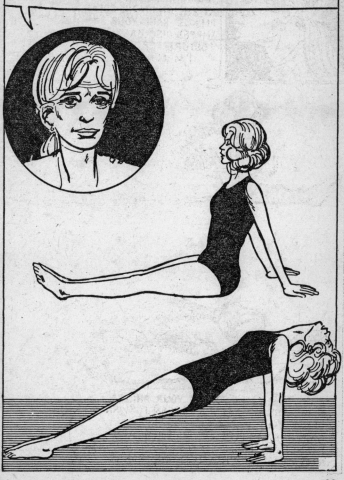

KAPOTASANA - Dove

KNEEL, STRETCH THE LEFT LEG OUT BEHIND YOU, AND SIT ON YOUR RIGHT HEEL. PUSHING OUT YOUR CHEST, LEAN RIGHT BACK AND EXTEND YOUR ARMS BEHIND YOU, PALMS OUTWARDS. ATTENTION IS FIXED ON THE BACK. TO LEAVE THE POSITION, LEAN FORWARDS. PUT YOUR FOREHEAD ON THE GROUND AND DRAW YOUR LEFT LEG BACK BESIDE YOUR RIGHT, WHICH YOU NOW STRETCH REARWARD TO REVERSE THE POSITION.

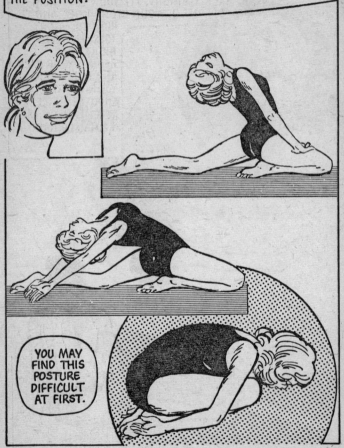

YOU MAY FIND THIS POSTURE DIFFICULT AT FIRST.

ARDHA MATSEYNDRASANA II — Complete twist

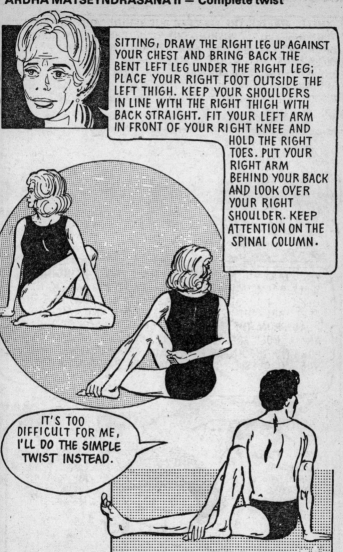

SITTING, DRAW THE RIGHT LEG UP AGAINST YOUR CHEST AND BRING BACK THE BENT LEFT LEG UNDER THE RIGHT LEG; PLACE YOUR RIGHT FOOT OUTSIDE THE LEFT THIGH. KEEP YOUR SHOULDERS IN LINE WITH THE RIGHT THIGH WITH BACK STRAIGHT. FIT YOUR LEFT ARM IN FRONT OF YOUR RIGHT KNEE AND HOLD THE RIGHT TOES. PUT YOUR RIGHT ARM BEHIND YOUR BACK AND LOOK OVER YOUR RIGHT SHOULDER. KEEP ATTENTION ON THE SPINAL COLUMN.

IT'S TOO DIFFICULT FOR ME, I'LL DO THE SIMPLE TWIST INSTEAD.

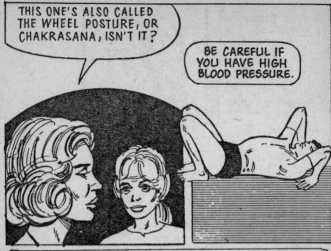

THIS ONE'S ALSO CALLED THE WHEEL POSTURE, OR CHAKRASANA, ISN'T IT?

BE CAREFUL IF YOU HAVE HIGH BLOOD PRESSURE.

YES. START ON THE BACK. BEND THE LEGS, BRINGING THE HEELS BACK TO THE BUTTOCKS; RAISE ELBOWS, HANDS UNDER SHOULDERS, FINGERS POINTING TOWARDS THE FEET. BREATHING IN, LIFT THE PELVIS AND RAISE THE HEAD FROM THE GROUND. KEEP ATTENTION ON THE ARMS. HOLD FOR 30 SECONDS, COME BACK SLOWLY, PUSHING THE KNEES FORWARD. THIS POSTURE TONES THE MUSCLES OF THE ABDOMINAL BELT AND BUILDS VITALITY.

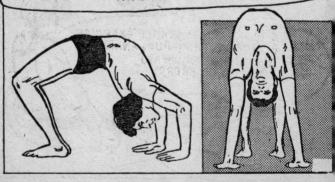

Balancing breathing

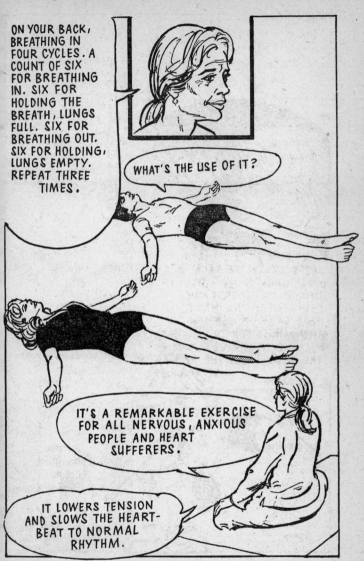

ON YOUR BACK, BREATHING IN FOUR CYCLES. A COUNT OF SIX FOR BREATHING IN. SIX FOR HOLDING THE BREATH, LUNGS FULL. SIX FOR BREATHING OUT. SIX FOR HOLDING, LUNGS EMPTY. REPEAT THREE TIMES.

WHAT'S THE USE OF IT?

IT'S A REMARKABLE EXERCISE FOR ALL NERVOUS, ANXIOUS PEOPLE AND HEART SUFFERERS.

IT LOWERS TENSION AND SLOWS THE HEART-BEAT TO NORMAL RHYTHM.

SUMMARY OF LESSON 4 FULL PRACTICE

1. Hero
   Bhadra

   Normal
   breathing,
   count 15-30
   each leg

2. Stretched
   triangle

   Normal
   breathing,
   count 30-60
   each side

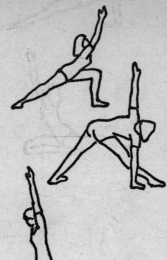

3. Squatting
   pose

   4-6 times

4. Relaxation

   2-3 mins

5. The sage

   1-2 mins

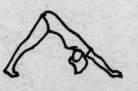

6. Dog pose

   Normal
   breathing,
   count 6
   Repeat 3 times

7. West
   stretch

   Hold for 6
   breaths, repeat
   3 times

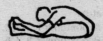

8. East stretch

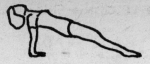

Hold for 3 breaths, repeat 3 times

9. Relaxation

1-2 mins

10. Dove

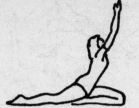

Hold for 3 breaths, 2 each leg

11. Half legendary hero

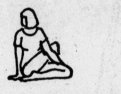

Normal breathing, count 30-60 each side

12. Arch in air

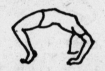

Normal breathing, count 20-60

13. Relax in devotion

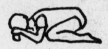

12 slow breaths

14. Balancing breath

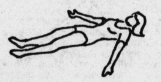

Breathe in/out and hold counting to 6. Repeat 3 times

Key posture: West stretch
Short practice — Day A: postures 1, 3, 4, 6, 7, 8, 5, 11, 13
Short practice — Day B: postures 2, 3, 4, 6, 7, 10, 9, 12, 14

Chapter 10

LESSON FIVE

By the time you reach this lesson you will probably have had ten weeks or so of practical experience in discovering yoga. You will be feeling much more supple with a lighter step. The way you move will feel more controlled and balanced and your breathing will be healthier. You should feel a pleasant sense of achievement in having improved your normal condition.

The West has more recently accepted, as yogis always have, that there is a close interrelation between body and mind, so close in fact that they are inseparable. You will find out that benefits affecting your physical system, bring about a corresponding improvement in your state of mind.

You will probably discover that you are taking a more relaxed attitude to life. There will be a stabilizing and calming effect on the mind. The demon, tension, which burdens so many people becomes easier to deal with. Relief from such pressures brings increased vitality and endurance. After all, yoga is a self-improvement course that has been developed over thousands of years.

Supine stretch

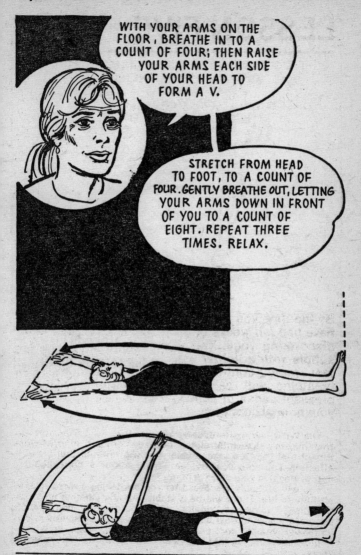

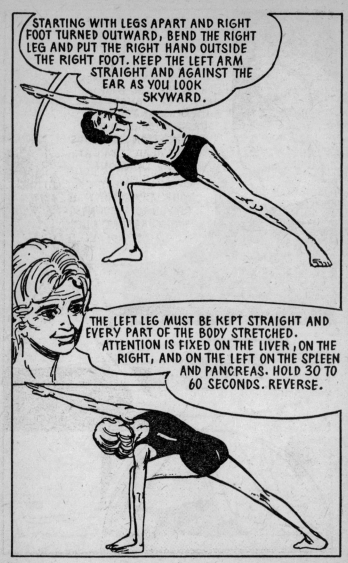

STARTING WITH LEGS APART AND RIGHT FOOT TURNED OUTWARD, BEND THE RIGHT LEG AND PUT THE RIGHT HAND OUTSIDE THE RIGHT FOOT. KEEP THE LEFT ARM STRAIGHT AND AGAINST THE EAR AS YOU LOOK SKYWARD.

THE LEFT LEG MUST BE KEPT STRAIGHT AND EVERY PART OF THE BODY STRETCHED. ATTENTION IS FIXED ON THE LIVER, ON THE RIGHT, AND ON THE LEFT ON THE SPLEEN AND PANCREAS. HOLD 30 TO 60 SECONDS. REVERSE.

PARSVOTTANASANA - Intense stretching of one side

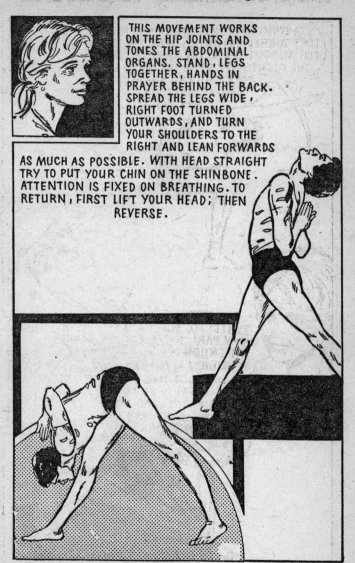

THIS MOVEMENT WORKS ON THE HIP JOINTS AND TONES THE ABDOMINAL ORGANS. STAND, LEGS TOGETHER, HANDS IN PRAYER BEHIND THE BACK. SPREAD THE LEGS WIDE, RIGHT FOOT TURNED OUTWARDS, AND TURN YOUR SHOULDERS TO THE RIGHT AND LEAN FORWARDS AS MUCH AS POSSIBLE. WITH HEAD STRAIGHT TRY TO PUT YOUR CHIN ON THE SHINBONE. ATTENTION IS FIXED ON BREATHING. TO RETURN, FIRST LIFT YOUR HEAD; THEN REVERSE.

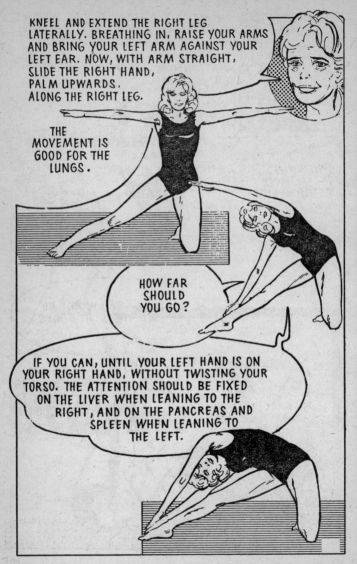

KNEEL AND EXTEND THE RIGHT LEG LATERALLY. BREATHING IN, RAISE YOUR ARMS AND BRING YOUR LEFT ARM AGAINST YOUR LEFT EAR. NOW, WITH ARM STRAIGHT, SLIDE THE RIGHT HAND, PALM UPWARDS, ALONG THE RIGHT LEG.

THE MOVEMENT IS GOOD FOR THE LUNGS.

HOW FAR SHOULD YOU GO?

IF YOU CAN, UNTIL YOUR LEFT HAND IS ON YOUR RIGHT HAND, WITHOUT TWISTING YOUR TORSO. THE ATTENTION SHOULD BE FIXED ON THE LIVER WHEN LEANING TO THE RIGHT, AND ON THE PANCREAS AND SPLEEN WHEN LEANING TO THE LEFT.

PARI PURNA NAVASANA - Complete boat

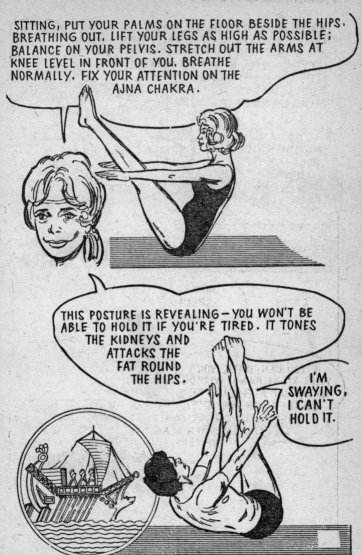

SITTING, PUT YOUR PALMS ON THE FLOOR BESIDE THE HIPS. BREATHING OUT, LIFT YOUR LEGS AS HIGH AS POSSIBLE; BALANCE ON YOUR PELVIS. STRETCH OUT THE ARMS AT KNEE LEVEL IN FRONT OF YOU. BREATHE NORMALLY. FIX YOUR ATTENTION ON THE AJNA CHAKRA.

THIS POSTURE IS REVEALING — YOU WON'T BE ABLE TO HOLD IT IF YOU'RE TIRED. IT TONES THE KIDNEYS AND ATTACKS THE FAT ROUND THE HIPS.

I'M SWAYING, I CAN'T HOLD IT.

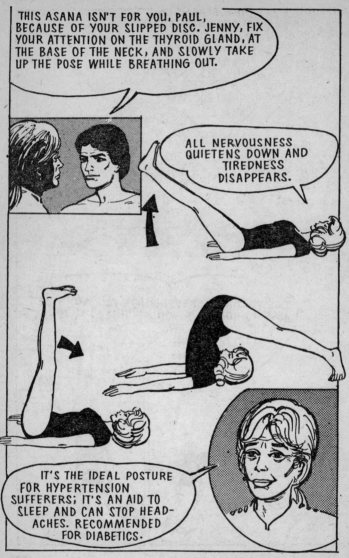

SHIRSASANA — Head-stand

KNEELING, PLACE THE FOREARMS ON THE FLOOR TO FORM A TRIANGLE AND INTERLOCK THE FINGERS TIGHTLY. WITH THE BACK OF THE HEAD IN THE CUPPED HANDS, AND WITHOUT MOVING THE FEET, RISE ON THE TOES AND PUSH UP THE PELVIS. DRAW THE FEET GENTLY TOWARDS THE FACE. WHEN YOU'VE FOUND YOUR BALANCE POINT, BEND YOUR LEGS AND LIFT THE HEELS TOWARDS THE PELVIS, THEN UP TOWARDS THE SKY. STRAIGHTEN YOUR LEGS AND YOU SHOULD FIND YOURSELF PERFECTLY BALANCED, THE WEIGHT RESTING ON THE ARMS.

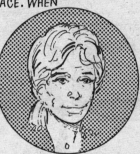

WARNING: DON'T TRY THIS ONE UNLESS YOUR CERVICAL VERTEBRAE ARE IN PERFECT CONDITION AND YOU HAVE NO CIRCULATION OR OVERWEIGHT PROBLEMS. IF IN DOUBT, IT IS ESSENTIAL THAT YOU CONSULT YOUR DOCTOR.

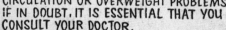

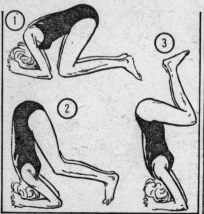

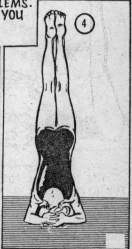

ALWAYS KEEP YOUR ATTENTION ON YOUR BACK. NOW RAISE BOTH YOUR LEGS BREATHING IN TO A COUNT OF FOUR; LUNGS FULL, HOLD THE POSITION. LOWER LEGS, BREATHING OUT TO A COUNT OF FOUR. PAUSE WITH LUNGS EMPTY.

DO I HAVE TO USE MY HANDS TO HELP ME?

LEAN ON YOUR CLOSED FISTS, IT WILL GIVE YOU MORE STRENGTH. AT FIRST YOU WON'T BE ABLE TO LIFT YOUR LEGS VERY FAR.

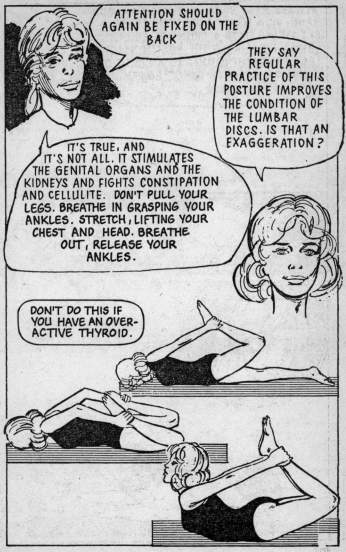

ATTENTION SHOULD AGAIN BE FIXED ON THE BACK

THEY SAY REGULAR PRACTICE OF THIS POSTURE IMPROVES THE CONDITION OF THE LUMBAR DISCS. IS THAT AN EXAGGERATION?

IT'S TRUE, AND IT'S NOT ALL. IT STIMULATES THE GENITAL ORGANS AND THE KIDNEYS AND FIGHTS CONSTIPATION AND CELLULITE. DON'T PULL YOUR LEGS. BREATHE IN GRASPING YOUR ANKLES. STRETCH, LIFTING YOUR CHEST AND HEAD. BREATHE OUT, RELEASE YOUR ANKLES.

DON'T DO THIS IF YOU HAVE AN OVER-ACTIVE THYROID.

UPAVISTA KONASANA - Sitting angle

SITTING, LEGS AS FAR APART AS POSSIBLE, TAKE THREE DEEP BREATHS FROM THE DIAPHRAGM. PUT YOUR HANDS ON YOUR THIGHS AND SLIDE THEM DOWN TO YOUR TOES, GRIPPING THE TOES. BEND FORWARD, BACK STRAIGHT, AND REST YOUR CHIN ON THE FLOOR. KEEP ATTENTION ON THE SOLAR PLEXUS. THIS POSTURE IS PARTICULARLY RECOMMENDED FOR WOMEN; IT HELPS THE CIRCULATION OF BLOOD IN THE PELVIC REGION AND EASES SCIATIC PAIN.

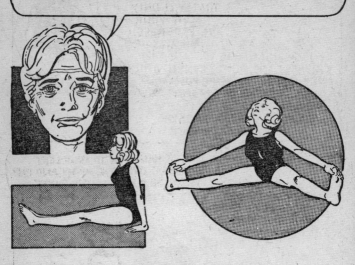

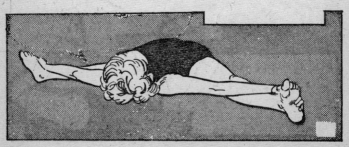

PADMASANA - Lotus

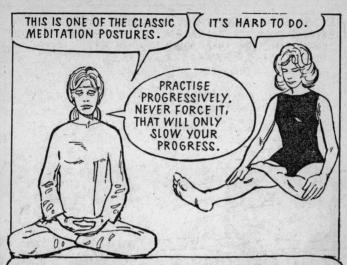

THIS IS ONE OF THE CLASSIC MEDITATION POSTURES.

IT'S HARD TO DO.

PRACTISE PROGRESSIVELY. NEVER FORCE IT, THAT WILL ONLY SLOW YOUR PROGRESS.

LIFT YOUR RIGHT FOOT WITH YOUR HANDS ON TO YOUR LEFT THIGH. TAKE THE LEFT FOOT, CROSS IT OVER THE RIGHT AND PUT IT ON THE RIGHT THIGH. PRACTISE A HALF LOTUS FIRST.

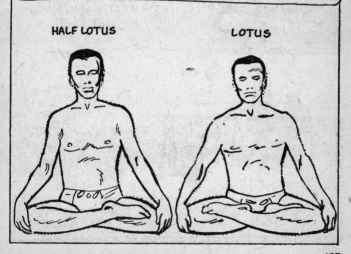

HALF LOTUS

LOTUS

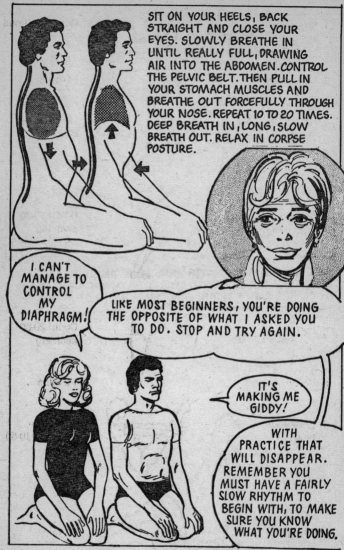

SIT ON YOUR HEELS, BACK STRAIGHT AND CLOSE YOUR EYES. SLOWLY BREATHE IN UNTIL REALLY FULL, DRAWING AIR INTO THE ABDOMEN. CONTROL THE PELVIC BELT. THEN PULL IN YOUR STOMACH MUSCLES AND BREATHE OUT FORCEFULLY THROUGH YOUR NOSE. REPEAT 10 TO 20 TIMES. DEEP BREATH IN, LONG, SLOW BREATH OUT. RELAX IN CORPSE POSTURE.

I CAN'T MANAGE TO CONTROL MY DIAPHRAGM!

LIKE MOST BEGINNERS, YOU'RE DOING THE OPPOSITE OF WHAT I ASKED YOU TO DO. STOP AND TRY AGAIN.

IT'S MAKING ME GIDDY!

WITH PRACTICE THAT WILL DISAPPEAR. REMEMBER YOU MUST HAVE A FAIRLY SLOW RHYTHM TO BEGIN WITH, TO MAKE SURE YOU KNOW WHAT YOU'RE DOING.

SUMMARY OF LESSON 5 FULL PRACTICE

1. Supine stretch 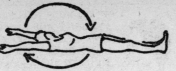 Repeat 3 times

2. Relaxation — 1-2 mins

3. Side triangle 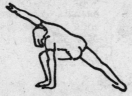 Count 20-60 each side

4. Intense stretching 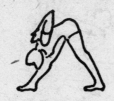 Count 10-30 each leg

5. Fence 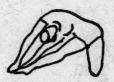 Count 20-60 each leg

6. Relaxation — 1-2 mins

7. Complete boat 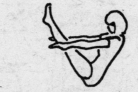 hold for a count of 10-50

8. Plough 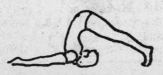 1-3 mins

9. Head stand 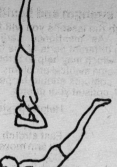 Count 30-60

10. Locust 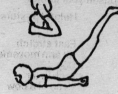 Repeat 3 times, relaxing front down in between

11. Relaxation front down 1-2 mins

12. Bow 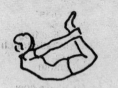 Count 10-60. Relax front down in between. Repeat 3 times

13. Sitting angle 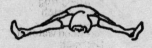 Try this gradually. Count 10-60

14. Lotus 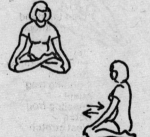 Try this gradually. 1-2 mins

15. Cleansing practice  20 cycles

16. Relaxation 1-2 mins

Key postures: Plough and Headstand
Short practice — Day A: postures 1, 3, 5, 8, 6, 10, 11, 14, 15
(Key posture: Plough)
Short practice — Day B: postures 1, 4, 7, 9, 6, 11, 13, 14, 15
(Key posture: Headstand)

Postures for strength and health

Working through the lessons you will feel more relaxed mentally and physically. As mentioned earlier, certain postures are associated with different parts of the body. Here is a quick guide to the postures which may help to strengthen various parts of the body and ease some medical problems.

Obviously all postures should be performed gently and, if you are in any doubt, consult your doctor.

Parts of the Body	Helpful postures	Lesson number
Shoulders, arms	East stretch	4
	All arm movements	
	Dog	4
	Arch in air	4
	Head of a cow	3
	Dove	4
Spinal column and muscles	Triangles	1
	Reverse	1
	Standing frog	2
	Back half-stretch	2
	Cobra	2
	Mountain	1
	Tree	2
	Head of a cow	3
	Kneeling frog	3
	West stretch	4
	Dove	4
	Reversed watcher	2
	Half arch	2
	Bow	5
	Locust	5
	Shoulder stand	3
	Head on knees	1
Back muscles	Half locust	1
	Staff	2
	Reversed watcher	2
	Half arch	2
	Standing frog	2
	Adept	3
	Kneeling frog	3
	Cobra	2
	West stretch	4
	Twisting	3
	Squatting	4
	Shoulder stand	3
Abdominal muscles	Torsion of abdomen	1
	Pillar	2
	Stork	3
	Boat	3
	Flying contraction	3
	Arch in the air	4

Parts of the body	Helpful postures	Lesson number
Abdominal organs	Torsion of abdomen	1
	Flying contraction	3
	Intense stretch	5
Liver and gall bladder	Big toes	2
	Shoulder stand	3
	West stretch	4
	Bow	5
	Cobra	2
	Arch in the air	4
	Flying contraction	3
	Fence	5
	Twisting	3 and 4
	Hero Bhadra	4
	Side triangle	5
Kidneys	Cobra	2
	Boat	3 and 5
	Shoulder stand	3
	Bow	5
	Locust	5
	Dog	4
Intestines	Intestinal passage	1
	Twisting	3
	Torsion of abdomen	1
Genital organs	Crocodile	3
	Boat	3
	Bow	5
Leg muscles	All standing poses	
	Dog	4
	Locust	5
	Bow	5
	West stretch	4
	Squatting	4
	Sitting angle	5
	Standing frog	2
	Pillar	2
Hamstrings	Back half-stretched	2
	Pillar	2
	Torsion of abdomen	1
	Twisting	3
	Locust	5
	Bow	5
	All standing poses	
	West stretch	4

Medical conditions	Helpful postures	Lesson number
Backache	see Back muscles	
Blood pressure: High	Corpse	1
	Ujjayi (reclining)	2
	Meditation	
	Sitting poses	
	West stretch	4
	Plough	5
	Alternate nostril (not holding breath)	3
Low	Sitting poses	
	Corpse	1
	Shoulder stand	3
	Plough	5
	West stretch	4
Breathing	Head on knees	1
	Mountain	1
	Ujjayi	2
	Complete breath	2
	Alternate nostril	3
	Cleansing practice	5
Constipation	All standing postures	
	Flying contraction	3
Colds, coughs, throat trouble	Reverse pose	1
	West stretch	4
	Big toes	2
	Ujjayi	2
Hyper-acidity, dyspepsia	see: Liver/gall bladder	
Headache	Devotion	2
	Corpse	1
	Plough	5
	Alternate nostril	3
	West stretch	4
	Shoulder stand	3
Heart trouble	Corpse	1
	Meditation	
	Ujjayi	2
	Alternate nostril	3
	Balancing breath	4

113

Medical conditions	Helpful postures	Lesson number
Insomnia	Cobra	2
	Corpse	1
	Shoulder stand	3
	West stretch	4
	Plough	5
	Alternate nostril	3
Indigestion	Torsion of abdomen	1
	Standing poses	
	Shoulder stand	3
	Flying contraction	3
	Locust	5
	Bow	5
	Twisting	3 and 4
Menstrual disorders (not during period)	Corpse	1
	Cobra	2
	Shoulder stand	3
	Stork	3
	Dog	4
	Sitting angle	5
	Flying contraction	3
	West stretch	4
Nerves/ tension	Corpse	1
	Complete breath	1
	Meditation	
	Balancing breath	4
	Plough	5
	Balance hold toe	3
	Ujjayi	2
	Alternate nostril	3
Sciatica	Torsion of abdomen	1
	West stretch	4
	Dog	4
	Bow	5
	Cobra	2
	Shoulder stand	3
	All standing poses	

Chapter 11

THE HEART OF YOGA

"Yoga is a calming of mental agitation", wrote the great master of yoga, Patanjali, in his celebrated Aphorisms, over 2000 years ago. The pathway to joy is opened to him whose mind is at peace.

The journey of this peace of mind starts with the physical postures which, as you have probably been finding, feel better and work better when given your full attention. When you are absorbed in asanas, they become meditation in movement, and it is this concentration together with relaxation which forms the heart of yoga. Total relaxation is achieved by relaxing the muscles in stages; breathing slows down and finally mental activity quietens down. The effectiveness of relaxation as a cure for tension and nervous problems is widely established.

Dharana

Mental concentration, Dharana, is the sixth Limb and may be developed as an exercise on its own: some of the methods are described in this chapter. The ability to clear the mind of agitation, slow the constant flow of thought and focus on the matter in hand, can be usefully applied to everyday activities. In yoga, the discipline is to keep the mind steadily fixed on considering a chosen object, to bring attention back when it wanders. In the meantime, the body functions safely but does not interfere at all.

Dhyana

The seventh Limb of yoga is Dhyana, meditation, a state in which one's thoughts are directed upon an object or thought, so as to form an unbroken flow, like the continuous pouring of oil from one vessel into another. This passes into the experience of Samadhi, the eighth Limb. Samadhi is reached at various levels and happens when the self-awareness is reduced to a minimum and the object or thought fills the consciousness. The knower and the known become one and there is a union with the Absolute, the universal Spirit.

Candle concentration

Place a lighted candle about three feet (1 metre) in front of you. Choose one of the sitting postures which we have been working on before, or use a chair. The main thing is to remain still and comfortable for some time, with the back and neck in line, sitting upright, and with the chin tucked in.

Gaze directly at the flame for about two minutes, blinking when necessary. Then close your eyes and press your palms lightly against them, keeping the flame as an image in your mind's eye view. Concentrate on the image and don't let it disappear. If it starts to fade away, simply bring it back by looking for it — with your eyes closed. Fix your mind on this image of the flame and let no other thoughts distract you. After one or two minutes put your hands back on your knees and relax. Once at a time is enough. You should find this a restful exercise.

Mental concentration — Visualisation

To concentrate by inwardly picturing an image, identify yourself with a rose. Close your eyes, this is an exercise of the imagination. It helps to be very precise in seeing the colour and shape of the rose, also to be aware of its scent and texture. When your mind wanders, bring it back again gently but firmly to the various aspects of the rose that you have been noticing. Then again, let go and sink your identity into awareness of the rose. This form of meditation can last four or five minutes.

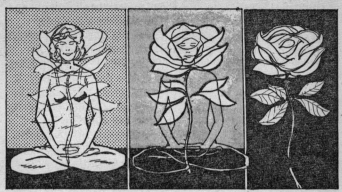

Try to picture a rose in your mind's eye

Mental concentration — Mantra, the yoga of sound

Group meditation, occasions of yoga discussions and learning often begin and end with the repetition of OM, uttered with a feeling of reverence. It is pronounced to rhyme with HOME, and is one of the greatest meditations. OM is a name for God and some of its uses are similar to the word AMEN.

If you choose to meditate on the sound of OM, the sacred Mantra, or incantation, repeat it to yourself inwardly or out loud, to the rhythm of your breathing, which will slow down by itself. Do this regularly, and in time you will attain a peaceful state of mind.

The Sanskrit symbol for OM

This is the Sanskrit symbol for OM. The long curve at the base represents a waking state. The shorter curve at the top half signifies dreamless sleep; and the curve drawn out from the junction represents the condition of dreaming. The state of liberation is represented in the semi-circle with the dot drawn above, since it is beyond the other three states — its incomplete circle is the symbol of infinity.

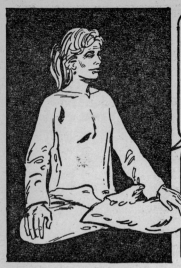

MENTALLY, INWARDLY, START EXAMINING YOUR BODY FROM THE SOLE OF THE RIGHT FOOT, SLOWLY, GOING UP ALONG THE LEG. MAKE SURE —FEEL—THAT THE ANKLE IS LOOSE AND HEAVY, AND THE KNEE JOINT, TOO. GO UP TO THE HIP JOINT; NOW ABANDON THE LEG WITH EVERY MUSCLE RELEASED. PASS ON TO THE LEFT FOOT AND SIMILARLY MOVE YOUR ATTENTION UP THE LEFT LEG, LETTING GO OF EVERY JOINT AND MUSCLE.

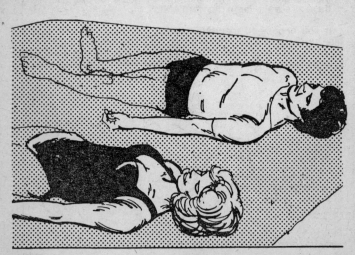

NOW MOVE THE FINGERS OF THE RIGHT HAND. RELEASE ALL TENSIONS... TAKE YOUR ATTENTION TO THE WRIST, THEN UP THE FOREARM TO THE ELBOW. GO UP TO THE SHOULDER JOINT; NOW ABANDON THE RIGHT ARM. PASS TO THE LEFT HAND, MAKE THE SAME PROGRESSION. ABANDON THE LEFT ARM.

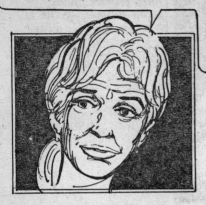

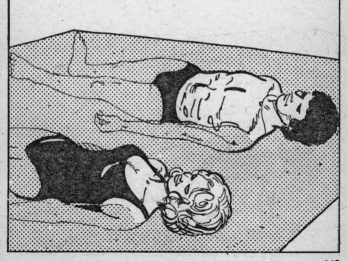

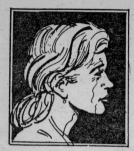

NOW START FROM THE BASE OF THE SPINE AND MOVE UP ALONG IT, RELAXING EACH MUSCLE ON THE WAY, ESPECIALLY IN THE NECK; THEN LOOSEN THE MUSCLES OF THE JAW, TONGUE AND THE FACIAL MUSCLES. THE EYELIDS SHOULD BE LIGHT, THE FOREHEAD AND SCALP RELAXED. YOUR BODY FEELS AS IF IT IS SINKING INTO THE EARTH. ALLOW A SMALL SMILE AT THE CORNERS OF YOUR MOUTH; YOU'RE FLOATING ON A CALM SEA, OR RESTING ON THE LAWN UNDER A BLUE SKY. STAY LIKE THIS FROM FIVE TO TEN MINUTES. THEN, STRETCHING FROM HEAD TO FOOT, BREATHE DEEPLY.

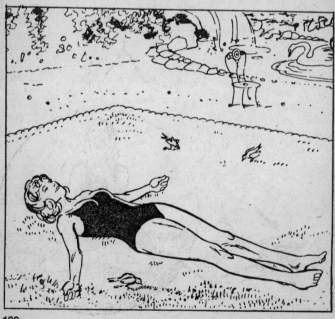

BEND YOUR LEGS GENTLY. ROLL OVER ON THE RIGHT SIDE AND PLACE YOUR LEFT HAND IN FRONT OF YOU TO LEAN ON; THEN SIT UP, LEGS CROSSED, TO PREPARE FOR THE BREATHING EXERCISE. CALLED NADI SODHANA, THIS TECHNIQUE CLEARS IMPURITIES FROM THE NADIS BEFORE YOU BEGIN MENTAL CONCENTRATION.

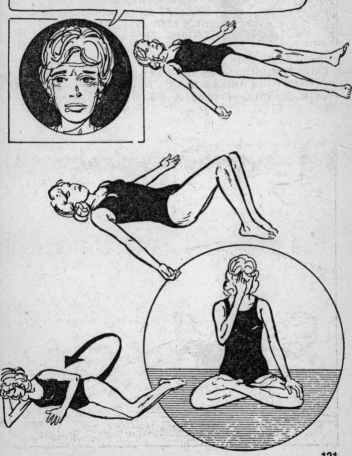

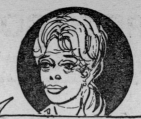

SIT ON THE EDGE OF A HARD CUSHION, THE HEIGHT DEPENDING ON YOUR PHYSIQUE. KNEES ON THE GROUND, SIT WITH SPINAL COLUMN PERFECTLY STRAIGHT AND CHIN SLIGHTLY DRAWN DOWN TO THE NECK. HANDS IN FRONT OF YOU, RIGHT ON LEFT, PALMS UPWARDS. SHUT YOUR EYES AND CONCENTRATE ON BREATHING. MENTALLY, INWARDLY, PRONOUNCE SO WHEN BREATHING IN, AHM WHEN BREATHING OUT. GENTLY, WITHOUT EFFORT, ALLOW YOUR MIND TO BECOME QUIET!

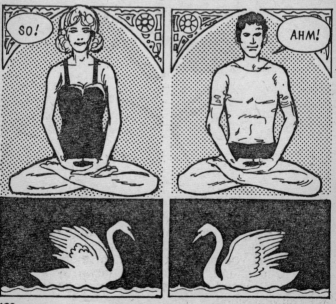

Chapter 12

WHERE TO GO
FROM HERE

As you near the end of this course of learning at home, it is a good idea to start looking at the world of yoga around you. You will find people with the same interests as you and amongst them there may be some who attend yoga classes taken by a yoga teacher. Weekend or day seminars on yoga are also held all year round.

By exploring in this way, you will find a teacher who suits you. Someone who can help you memorise postures by taking you through them regularly in class, and who can check that you are doing them correctly. You will have wondered before now whether you are doing the postures correctly and whether you are making progress. Joining a class for a while can help to answer your questions.

There are many sorts of teachers, all working in different ways and at different levels, as yoga is a living science that is growing all the time. Up and down the country there are Adult Education Centres which have day and evening yoga classes. You could also enquire at the British Wheel of Yoga which is an association organised on a regional basis throughout the country and is in touch with private classes, as well as the Adult Education Centres.

Reading about Yoga

If you want know what's going on in the yoga world, there is a monthly magazine called *Yoga Today*, which will give you information and ideas.

If you want to go further into the philosophy of yoga, you may like to read the ancient books written about yoga.

One, already mentioned in Chapter 3, is the writing of Pantanjali, which sets down 196 Sutras (or short statements) on various aspects of yoga, including the structure and stages of yoga (the eight limbs) and the ideas behind it.

Another ancient text which you may find interesting to read is the Upanishads. Upanishad means "sitting at the feet of a master". The Upanishads are sacred texts which form part of the Vedas, the oldest writings of India. No one knows who were the scholars, poets and mystics who wrote the Upanishads, but they were composed between 800 and 400 B.C., with a few additions made up until the fifteenth century A.D. If all the Upanishads were collected together in one volume, it would be about as long as the Bible.

These inspired revelations concern the nature of man and the universe and the union of the soul with the Absolute. Modern versions of the Upanishads usually deal with selections from 12 of the Upanishads.

Finally there is the Bhagavad Gita, which means "Song of God" or "Celestial Song" and is about 2000 years old. It is an epic poem of 700 verses, which is made up of a dialogue between two heroes of the warrior caste. They are on the field of battle, which can be regarded as the symbolic struggle between good and evil. One, the charioteer, is Krishna, a god among men and from the darker folk who originally inhabited India, and the other is Prince Arjuna, a fair-skinned descendent of the Aryan invaders who brought the horse to India. The horse is a symbol which appears frequently.

The Bhagavad Gita ranges across a host of ideas and explanations about yoga. It defines many kinds of yoga and recommends a common sense approach to yoga.

All these books are easily available in paperback translations with helpful commentaries.

GLOSSARY

Absolute: See Brahman.

Ananda: Perfect bliss, transcendental joy.

Asana: Posture.

Bhagavad Gita: "The Song of God", or "The Celestial Song". Celebrated scripture which formulates in poetic and dramatic form the basic mystical philosophy in yoga.

Bhakti Yoga: The yoga of love, devotion and submission to the will of the Absolute.

Brahman or Absolute: The supreme Reality which is one and indivisible, infinite, outside which no other reality exists. Universal Being that is beyond intellectual concepts and can only be comprehended by becoming one with it in the highest state of consciousness.

Buddhi: Reason, intelligence, power of understanding.

Chakra: Centre, wheel. The six psychic centres through which energy flows in the subtle body:

    Muladhara: Centre at the base of the spine;

    Svadhisthana — Abdominal centre;

    Manipura — Umbilical centre;

    Anahata — Heart centre;

    Vishuddha — Throat centre;

    Ajna — Centre between the eyebrows.

Citta: (pronounced CHITTA): That part of the spirit containing intelligence, ego, and sense-perception.

Dharana: Concentraton, total attention on an object or idea.

Dhyana: Meditation. Continuous effort of awareness to understand the object of concentration.

Guru: Spiritual guide and master.

Hatha-Yoga: Yoga proceeding principally by means of the physical body.

Jiva: Life. The core of pure consciousness.

Jnana: Metaphysical knowledge.

Jnana Yoga: Yoga which proceeds by means of Jnana.

Karma: Action. Spiritual cause and effect. Every action, good or bad, has its consequences which we cannot avoid.

Karma Yoga: The Yoga of selfless action in the world.

Kundalini or Kundalini-Shakti: The energy ("Serpent Power") imprisoned in the Muladhara Chakra at the base of the spine. It can be liberated by yoga. Penetrating into Sushumna (the central Nadi) it then joins cosmic consciousness in the Sahasrara, the thousand-petalled lotus at the top of the head; the Yogi then attains Samadhi, or enlightenment.

Kurma: Turtle or tortoise.

Manas: The higher part of mind which generates and controls intellect and such qualities as love, altruism and harmonious co-operation with others.

Mantra: A word or syllable with spiritual potential; a sound which is repeated to produce a lift of consciousness.

Maya: Cosmic illusion; the world of appearances, of relativity and duality.

Moksha: Spiritual liberation from the ego; liberation from the need to re-incarnate.

Nirvana: Extinction of the individual self as a separate being. Enlightenment. Immersion of the individual self in the infinity of existence.

OM or AUM: original sound representing supreme spiritual Reality. Sacred syllable. Used at the beginning and end of a recital of scripture or invocation, or at the beginning of scripture or invocation, or at the beginning of meditation to raise the level of consciousness.

Prajna: Spiritual wisdom.

Prakriti: The source of nature. Material cause of the universe.

Prana: Vital energy; vital breath; dynamism linking mind to matter.

Pranayama: Yoga techniques of breath control.

Pratyahara: Withdrawal of the mind from objects and the senses.

Rishi: Spiritual master, enlightened sage.

Sadhak or Sadhaka: One who practises the discipline of Yoga.

Sadhana: Spiritual practice or quest.

Samadhi: Superconscious, ecstatic state of union with ultimate reality. See Nirvana.

Samskaras: Fixed mental formations, impression of old habits or experience accumulated in the subconscious. Memories that remain.

Samyama: The three stages of the meditation process in Raja-Yoga comprising: Dharana — concentration; Dhyana — contemplation; Samadhi — ecstasy.

Sannyasin: One who has renounced the world. A Hindu aspirant who has taken on the fourth stage of life and renounced all worldly goods and desires and the privileges of caste. Often leads a wandering life, learning, teaching and helping others when he can.

Sat: Character of what is; existing; being; real, essential; true; beautiful; the infinite.

Shakti: Cosmic energy or power.

Shanti: Peace.

Siddha: He who has achieved spiritual perfection in himself.

Sukshma Sharira: The subtle body.

Tapas: Purificatory act, or preparation of the body. Heat, or ardour; often used to indicate excess. Exaggerated austerity, asceticism, mortifications. Leads to physical and sensory powers.

Turiya: State of consciousness including but transcending waking, dreaming, deep sleep; synonym of Samadhi.

Upanishads: A collection of philosophical and spiritual writings that were added to the Vedas. They are concerned with the nature of man and the universe and the union of soul and Absolute.

Vedas: Ancient Aryan scriptures of India, the earliest composed about 2,500 BC. There are four: **Rig-Veda, Sama-Veda, Yajur-Veda, Atharva-Veda.**

Vedanta: The basic mystical philosophy from which spring Yoga and the other doctrines of Hinduism.

Vidya: The science of principles; metaphysics.

Viveka: Just discrimination; discernment.

Vritti: Mental flux, that is to say, an idea. There are five kinds: exact knowledge, wrong knowledge, memories, dreams, imagination.